Adegboyega Akere MD, FWACP, DTMH, FRSTMH, Cert. Gastro & GI Endoscopy, MACG
Senior Lecturer & Consultant Physician & Gastroenterologist
Dept. of Medicine, College of Medicine,
University of Ibadan & University College Hospital,
Ibadan, Nigeria.

Jesse Abiodun Otegbayo MBBS, MSc, PhD, Cert. Gastro. FWACP, FACG, FRCP
Professor & Consultant Physician & Gastroenterologist
Dept. of Medicine, College of Medicine,
University of Ibadan & University College Hospital,
Ibadan, Nigeria.

Foreword

Since the first use of a straight rigid tube for gastroscopy about 150 years ago, upper gastrointestinal endoscopy has really come a long way. Transiting from the rigid through the semi-flexible and to the current flexible video endoscopes, the direct visualization of the gastrointestinal tract (GIT) has not only become feasible, a wide range of therapeutic interventions are now being done by endoscopy.

The earliest known fibreoptic GIT endoscopic studies in Nigeria were carried out in the early 1970s, close to 30 years after their introduction in Europe and America. For a long time, the procedure remained available only in a few scattered centres in the country due mainly to grossly inadequate trained manpower for endoscopy and unaffordability of the procedure by most Nigerians. Happily, the situation has begun to change with more centres in different parts of Nigeria now offering a wide range of endoscopic services, both diagnostic and therapeutic.

The authors who are active members and resource persons for the Society for Gastroenterology & Hepatology in Nigeria (SOGHIN) have produced an excellent book on upper gastrointestinal endoscopy which is, arguably, the first of its kind not only in Nigeria but also in the West African sub-region.

The book details the pictorial anatomy and annotated illustration of the most known lesions of the upper gastrointestinal tract right from the epiglottis to the second part of the duodenum. The clarity and the orderliness of the presentations are highly commendable. Resident doctors wanting to specialize in Gastroenterology and Endoscopy and practising Consultant Gastroenterologists who desire to enhance their diagnostic capabilities will find this book valuable.

Professor Dennis A. Ndububa MB, BS, FWACP, AGAF
Obafemi Awolowo University Teaching Hospital, Ile-Ife, Nigeria
July 2017

Preface

Since the introduction of gastrointestinal endoscopy, diagnosis of gastrointestinal diseases has become easier. Over the years, endoscopy equipment had undergone several modifications for better performance and efficiency. In order to gain maximum benefit from these equipment, the endoscopist must be able to recognize normal findings, as well as diagnose different abnormalities that can occur in the gastrointestinal tract.

This atlas contains different endoscopic pictures ranging from normal findings to a wide range of abnormalities. The pictures contained in this atlas were taken from patients who underwent endoscopy at our centre. There is a short description preceding the pictures for easy understanding.

This atlas will be of use to medical and surgical resident doctors in training, newly qualified specialists, other doctors with special interest in gastrointestinal endoscopy, as well as medical students. It is therefore hoped that, this book would be of help to our readers.

Adegboyega Akere

Acknowledgements

I thank the Almighty God for making this book a reality. I thank Him for the inspiration, wisdom and strength He gave to me to be able to write this book.

I want to thank the Chief Medical Director of the University College Hospital, Ibadan, Prof. T.O. Alonge for his efforts in providing the state-of-the-art Olympus endoscopy equipment which made the acquisition and compilation of the pictures in this atlas possible and easy.

Prof. J.A. Otegbayo was the CMAC/Director of Clinical Services when these equipment were acquired. He contributed immensely to make the purchase of these particular equipment possible.

I thank the Provost, College of Medicine, Prof. B.L. Salako for his advice and support. I thank my HOD, Prof. A.O. George for his support.

I also thank my wife, Olajumoke Modupe Akere and our children, Oluwadabira and Omotayo Akere for their support and encouragement during the preparation of this atlas.

My appreciation also goes to the following people for their support in one way or the other to the success of this book:

- Dr. K.O. Akande - Consultant Physician & Gastroenterologist
- Dr. T.O. Oke – Senior Registrar, Gastroenterology Unit
- Dr. Tinuola Fakoya - Senior Registrar, Gastroenterology Unit
- Dr. E.A. Tejan - Senior Registrar, Gastroenterology Unit
- Mrs. Stella Ayinde – Chief Nursing Officer, Endoscopy Unit
- Mrs. Eunice Akeju - Chief Nursing Officer, Endoscopy Unit
- Mrs. Modupe Isiaka - Chief Nursing Officer, Endoscopy Unit
- Mrs. Victoria Idowu – Assistant Chief Nursing Officer, Endoscopy Unit
- Miss Yetunde Ogunkunle – Assistant Chief Nursing Officer, Endoscopy Unit
- Mrs. Rahila Gashau – Nursing Officer, Endoscopy Unit
- Mrs. Omolola Afolagboye - Nursing Officer, Endoscopy Unit
- All the support members of staff of Endoscopy Unit

Contents

		Pages
1.	Authors	1
2.	Foreword	2
3.	Preface	3
4.	Acknowledgements	4
5.	Contents	5
6.	Introduction	6
7.	Epiglottis, Larynx & Oropharynx	7-10
8.	Oesophageal opening	11-12
9.	Normal Oesophagus	13-23
10.	Oesophageal Abnormalities	24-49
11.	Normal Stomach	50-62
12.	Gastric Abnormalities	63-85
13.	Normal Duodenum	86-92
14.	Duodenal Abnormalities	93-102
15.	References	103

CHAPTER 1

INTRODUCTION

Upper gastrointestinal endoscopy is also referred to as Oesophagogastroduodenoscopy (OGD). The term endoscopy is derived from two Greek words: endo (within) and skopein (to view or observe). Early efforts to visualize the human body orifices dated back to Egyptian and Greco-Roman times. Philip Bozzini was the first to examine the interior of a human body using a primitive endoscope in 1805. However, the first gastroscopy with a rigid endoscope was performed in 1868 by Adolf Kussmaul.

After these initial attempts, gastrointestinal endoscopes had undergone several stages of development through semi-flexible scopes to fibreoptics, and to the present day videoscopes.

During OGD, the oesophagus, stomach and down to the second part of the duodenum are usually visualized. A forward viewing gastroscope is often employed for this purpose. Before the procedure, the oropharynx is usually sprayed with 2% xylocaine as a form of local anaesthesia. The patient is also given "conscious sedation" with either intravenous diazepam or midazolam. Sometimes, low dose intravenous analgesics like, pentazocine or pethidine is given in addition.

Basically, there are 2 ways of intubating the oesophagus: the "blind" approach and under direct vision. However, direct vision is advocated because it allows inspection of the larynx and the oropharynx.

CHAPTER 2

The Normal Epiglottis, Larynx and Oropharynx

The vocal cords are visible and their movement can be assessed by asking the patient to say "aa"

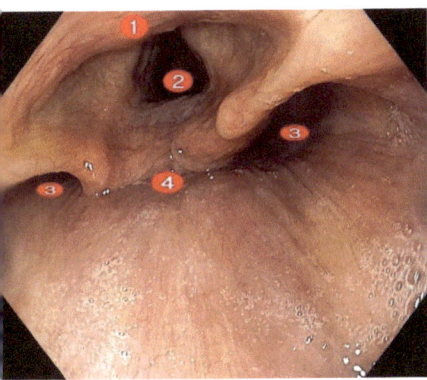

Figure 2.1

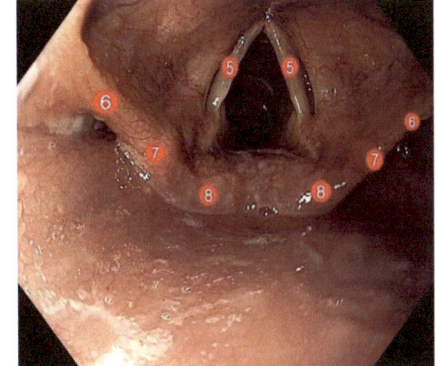

Figure 2.2

1. Valleculae
2. Trachea
3. Piriform sinuses
4. Oesophageal inlet

5. Vocal folds
6. Aryepiglottic fold
7. Cuneiform cartilage
8. Corniculate cartilage

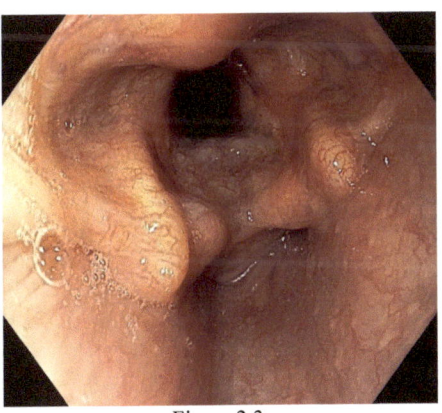

Figure 2.3

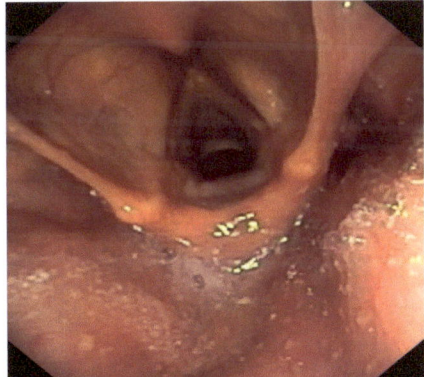

Figure 2.4

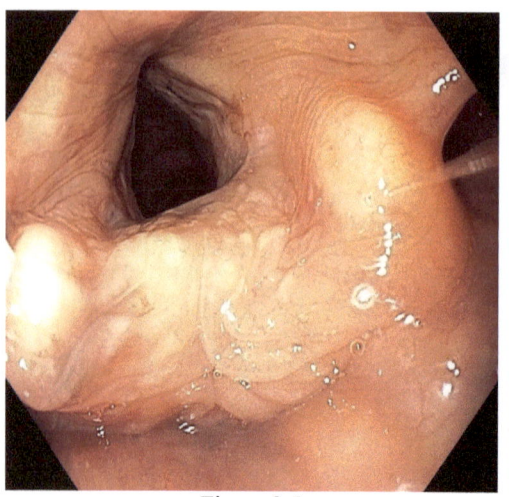
Figure 2.5

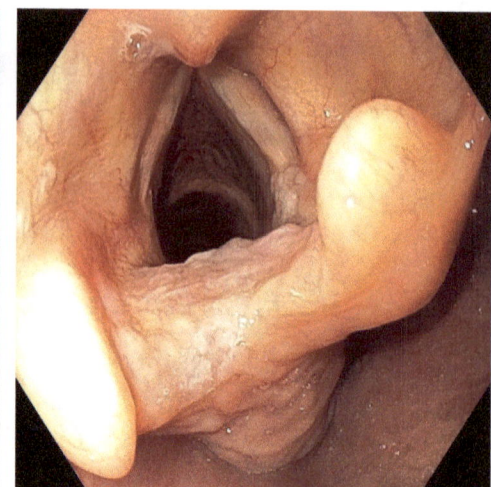
Figure 2.6

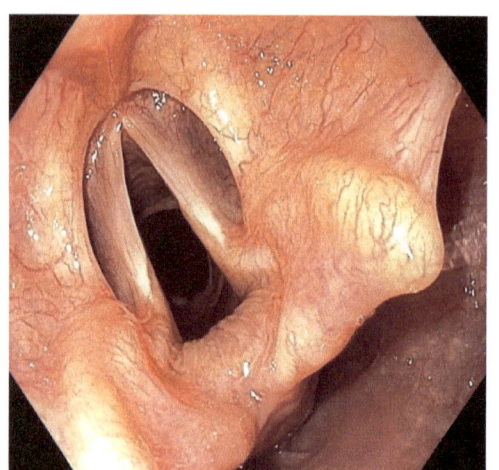
Figure 2.7

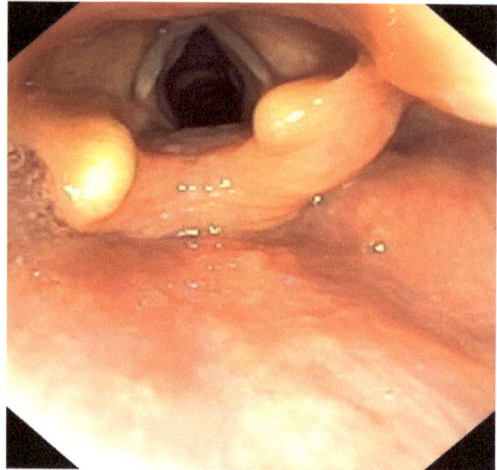
Figure 2.8

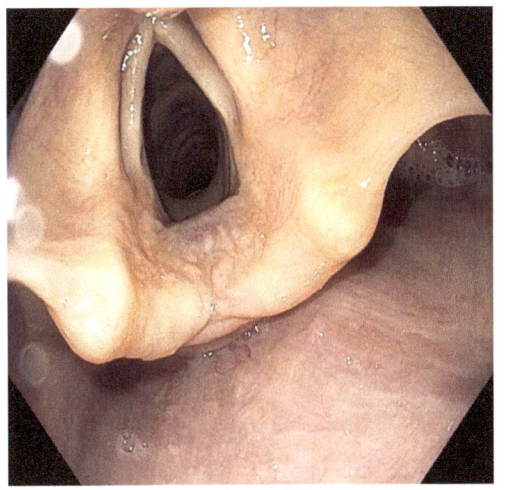

Figure 2.9

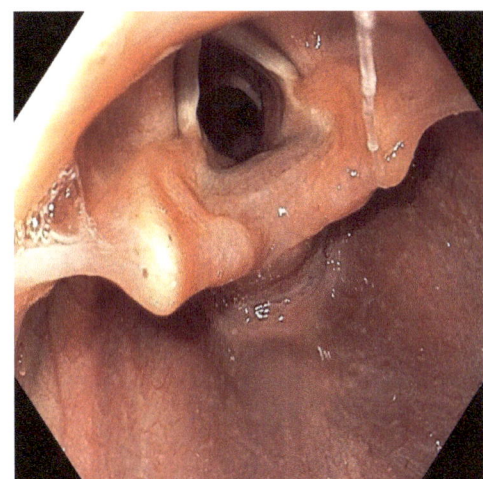

Figure 2.10

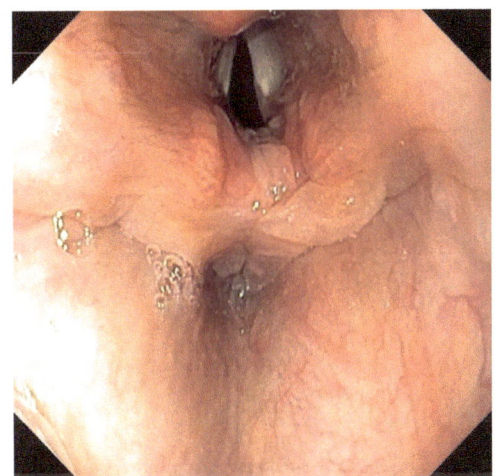

Figure 2.11

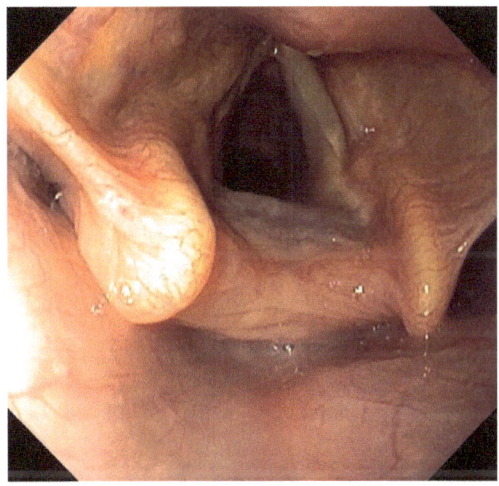

Figure 2.12

The epiglottis closes the airways to prevent aspiration during swallowing. In the resting position, it is usually thrown forward.

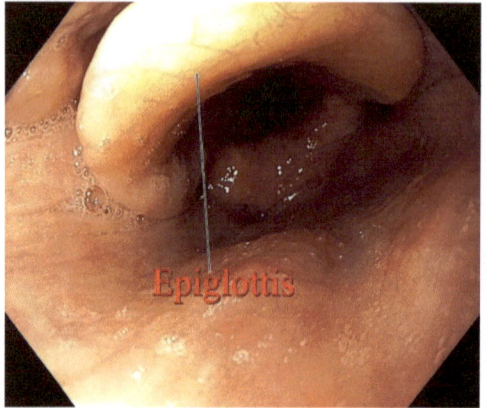

Figure 2.13

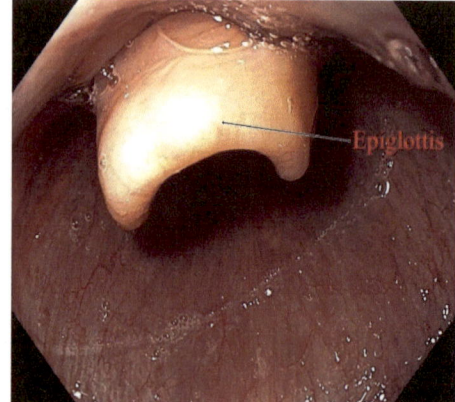

Figure 2.14

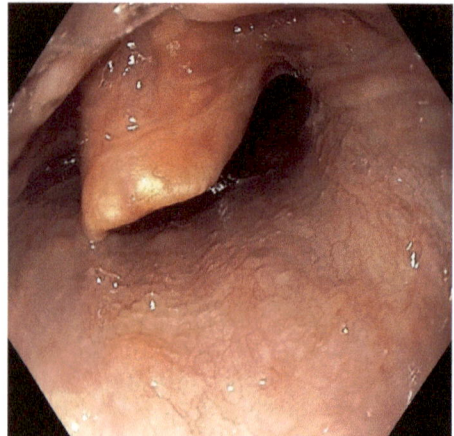

Figure 2.15

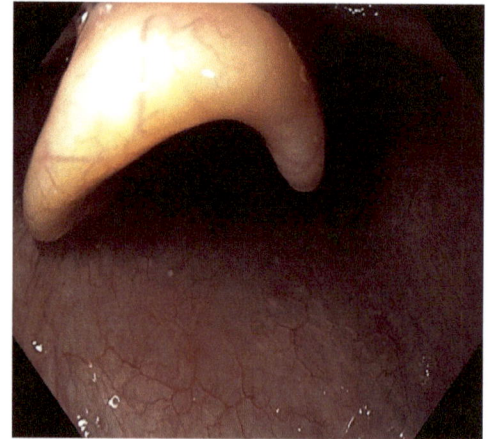

Figure 2.16

The oesophageal opening (inlet) is usually closed, and on each side of it, are the piriform fossae. When the patient is asked to swallow, the oesophageal opening (cricopharyngeal sphincter) opens and allows introduction of the endoscope

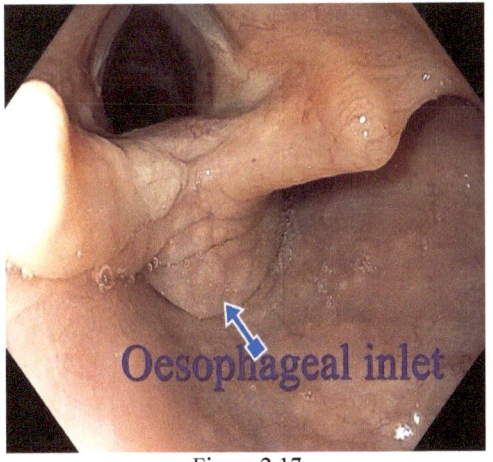

Figure 2.17

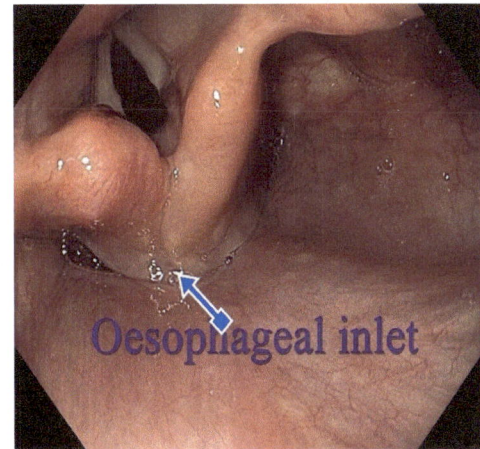

Figure 2.18

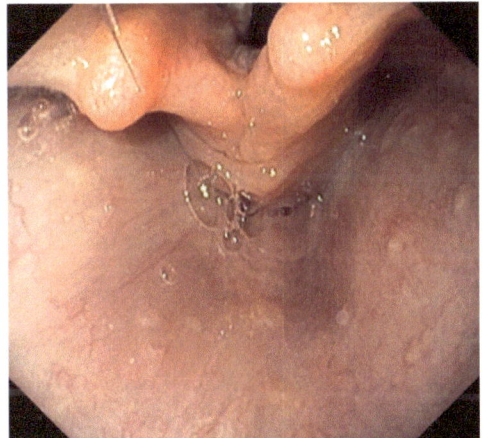

Figure 2.19

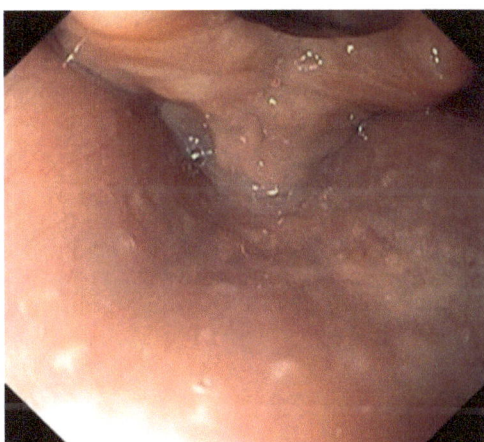

Figure 2.20

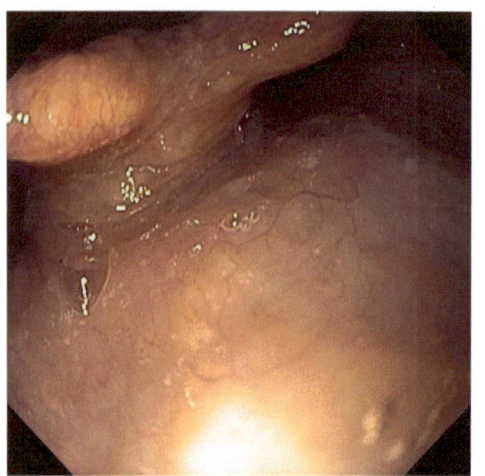
Figure 2.21

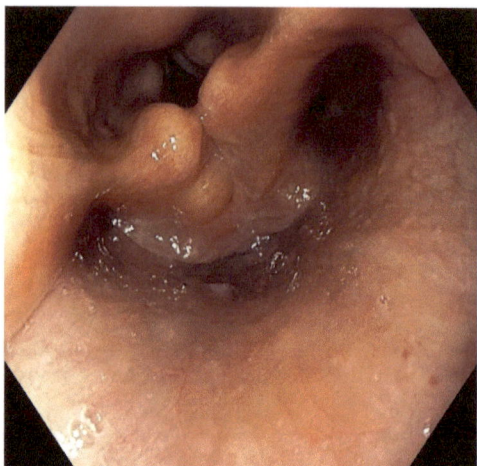
Figure 2.22

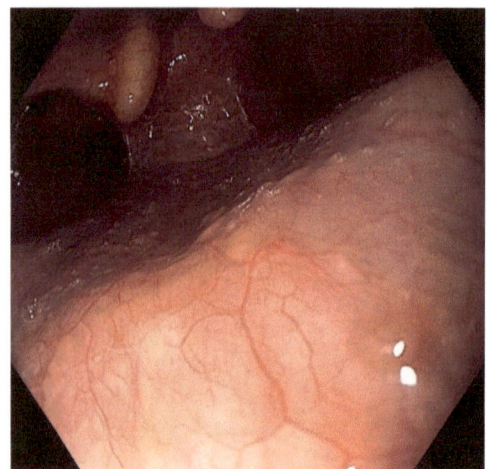
Figure 2.23

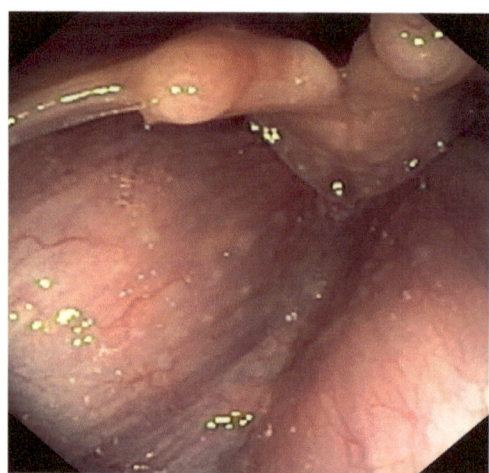
Figure 2.24

CHAPTER 3
The oesophagus

The oesophagus is a tube-like structure that serves as a conduit for food. The measurement of the length of the oesophagus is usually done in relation to the incisor teeth. Although, its actual length is about 20-24 cm and it begins at about 14-16 cm distal to the incisor teeth at the cricopharyngeus. So, in relation to the incisor teeth, the lowest level of the oesophagus where it enters the stomach is at about 34-40 cm.

The different parts of the oesophagus are:
- The upper oesophageal sphincter (UES)
- The cervical oesophagus
- The middle oesophagus
- The lower oesophagus

The middle and the lower parts make up the thoracic oesophagus

The UES is the first part and entrance to the oesophagus. It is a high pressure zone and usually relaxes when the patient is asked to swallow, thereby allowing the scope to pass through. The mucosa is smooth and reddish-gray in colour. Underneath the mucosa, superficial longitudinal venous plexuses are visible.

The cervical oesophagus is straight, featureless, round and symmetrical tube of about 6cm in length.

The midoesophagus is about 27 cm from the incisors. Here, indentations from adjacent organs can be seen in the lumen. These include: indentations of the spinal column at 12 0'clock, the left main bronchus at 6 0'clock, the left atrium and the aortic arch laterally which runs horizontally and is proximal, and on the right to the bronchus.

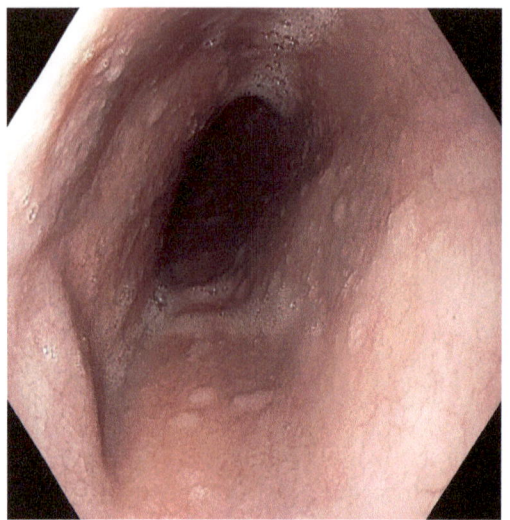

Figure 13.1

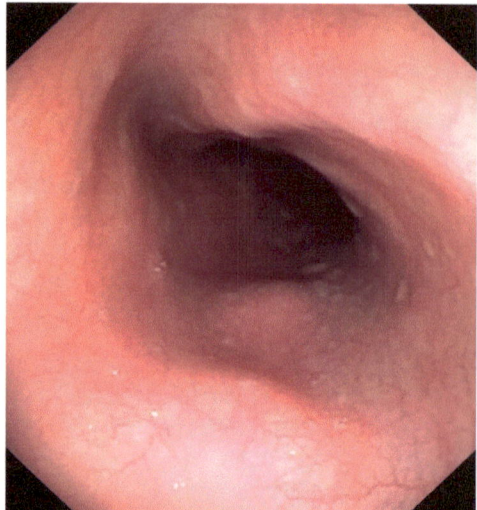

Figure 13.2

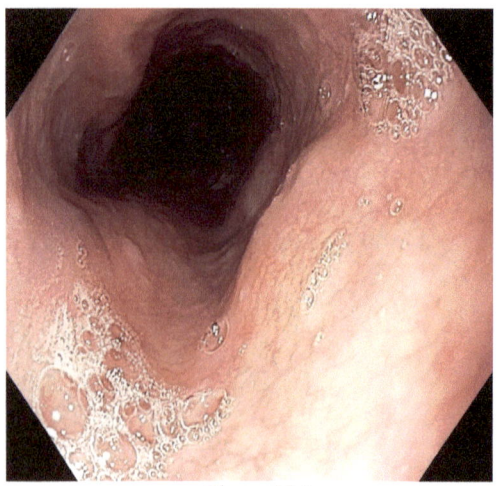

Figure 13.3

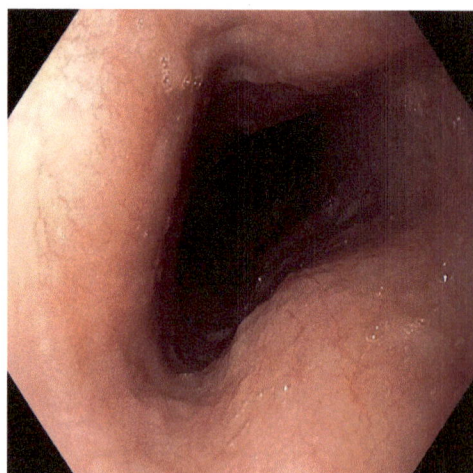

Figure 13.4

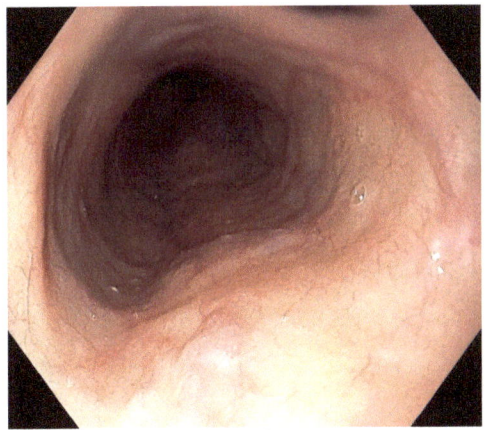 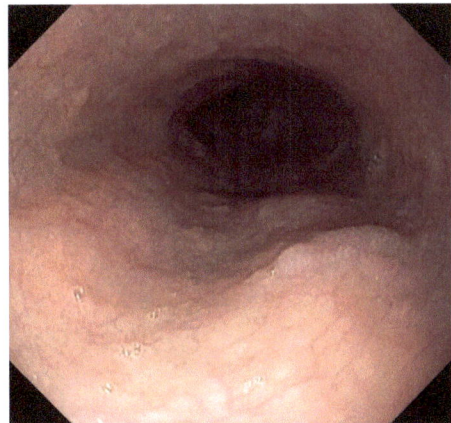

Figure 13.5   Figure 13.6

At about 30-38 cm from the incisors, there is a portion of the oesophagus called retrocardiac oesophagus, which has elliptical lumen due to compressions from the left atrium and aorta. Here, distinct pulsations of the heart can be visible and very useful for Transoesophageal Echocardiography.

The distal oesophagus is about 36-38 cm from the incisors. Characteristics of this region are the lower oesophageal sphincter (LES) and external pressure from the diaphragmatic crura. Here, longitudinal folds with concentric luminal narrowing can be seen as a result of muscular contraction and the underlying venous plexus.

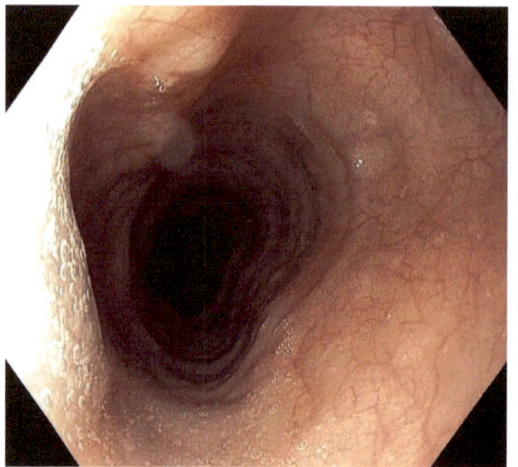

Figure 13.7
Here, some concentric rings are visible in the lumen. This is a normal finding, especially when the lumen is not fully distended.

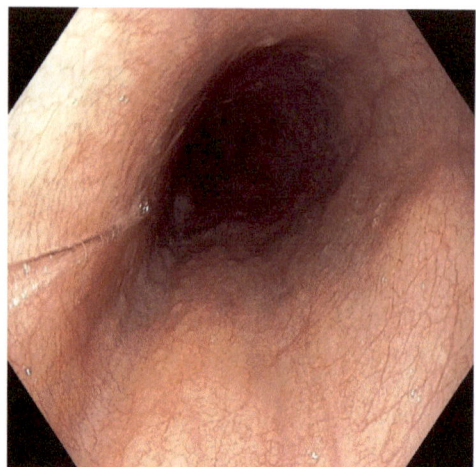

Figure 13.8

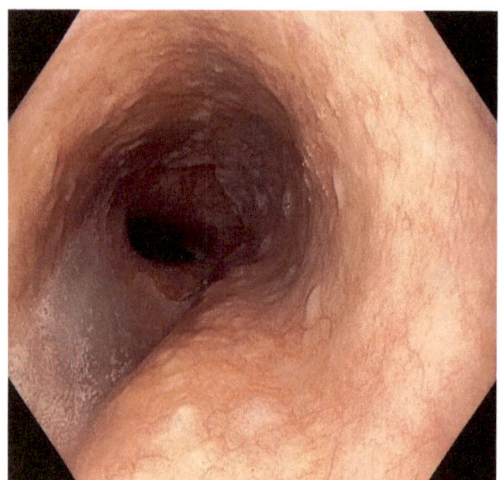

Figure 13.9

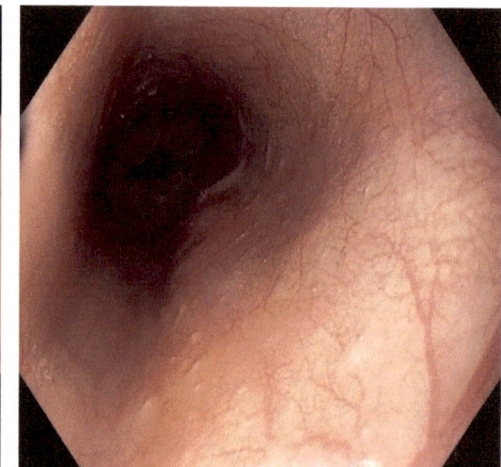

Figure 13.10

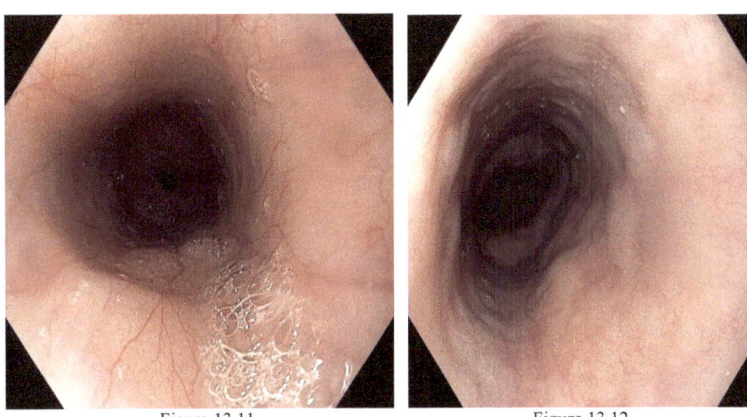

Figure 13.11

Figure 13.12

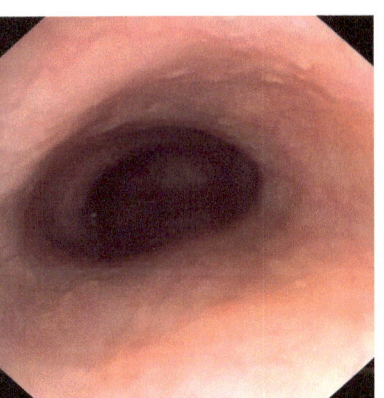

Figure 13.13

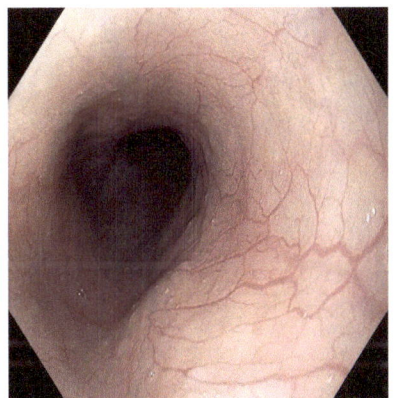

Figure 13.14
The fine vascular network of the oesophagus is depicted here. This is a normal finding.

Gastroesophageal Junction

Gastroesophageal junction (GEJ) is also called squamocolumnar junction, dentate or Z-line. It is about 35-41 cm from the incisors. It is complex, both anatomically and functionally. It represents the junction between the oesophageal squamous epithelium (pale-pink or gray in colour) and the stomach columnar epithelium (red and slightly raised). This junction has variable appearance and this includes:
- Indistinct
- Ring-shaped
- Jagged
- Flame-shaped
- Finger-like proximal extension of gastric mucosa
- Islands of gastric mucosa surrounded by oesophageal mucosa, and vice versa

Indistinct Z-line

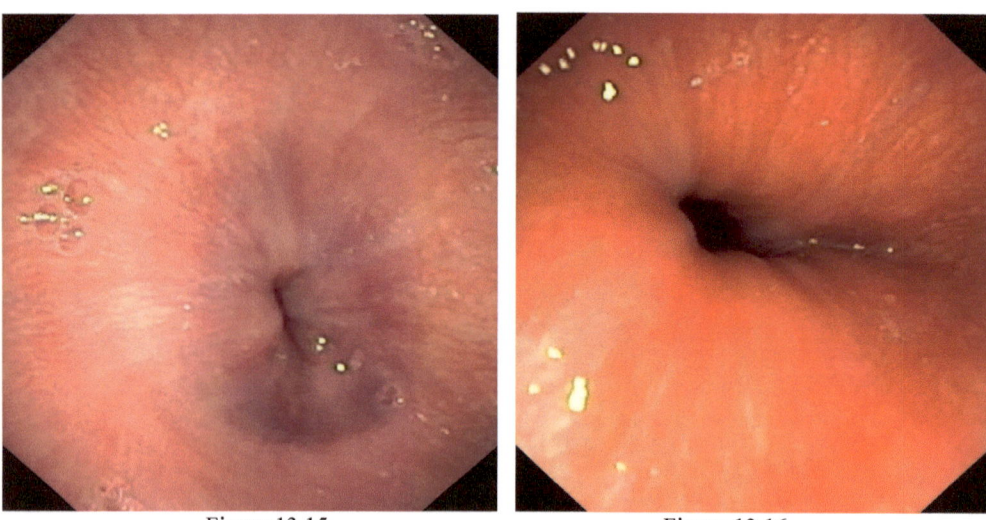

Figure 13.15   Figure 13.16

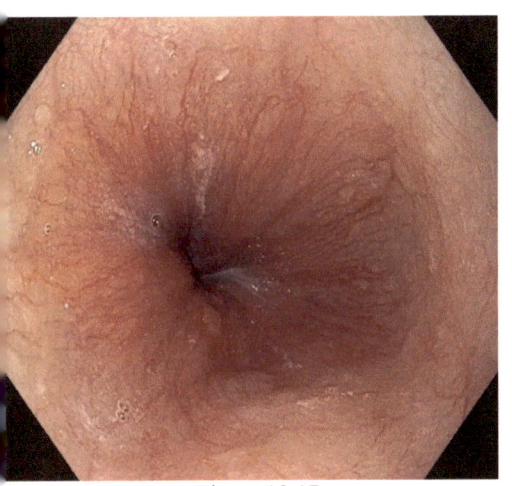

Figure 13.17

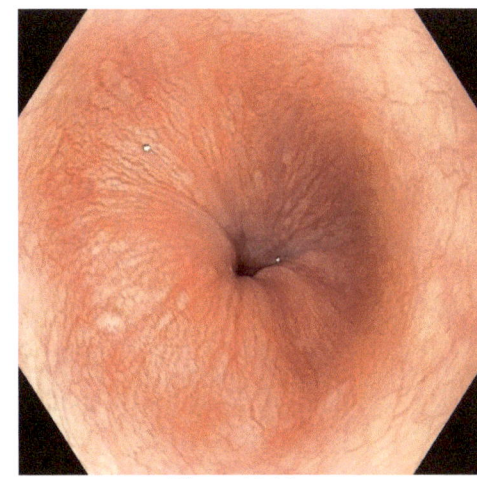

Figure 13.18

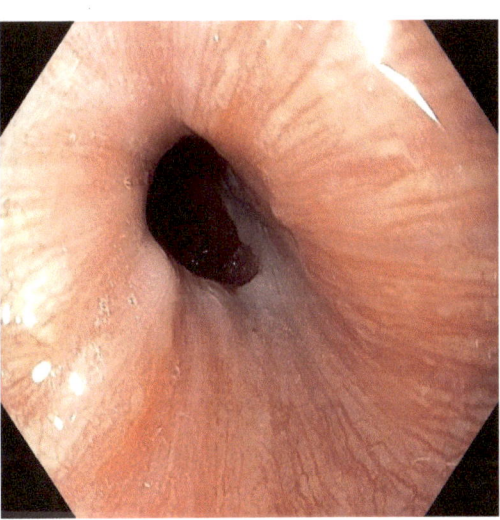

Figure 13.19

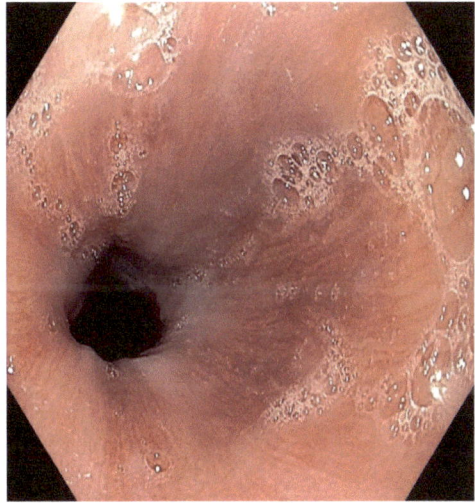

Figure 13.20

Ring-shaped Z-line

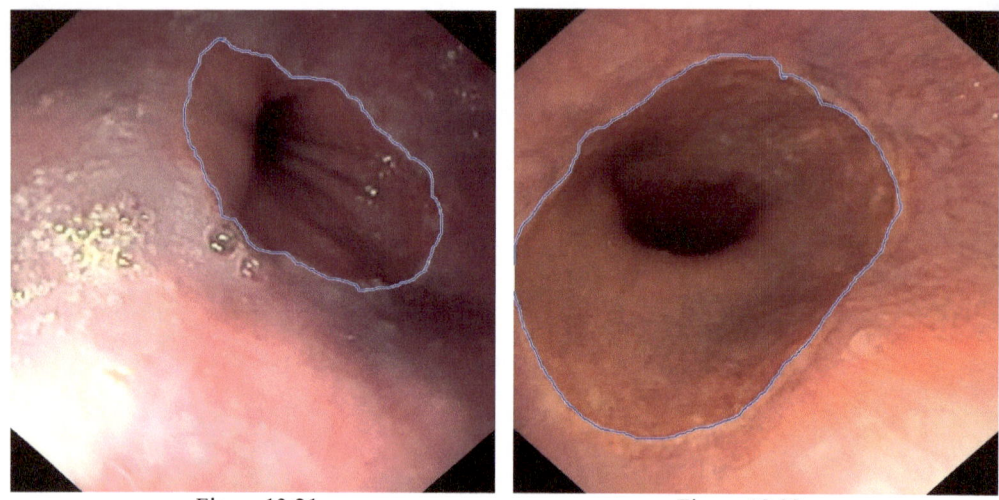

Figure 13.21

Figure 13.22

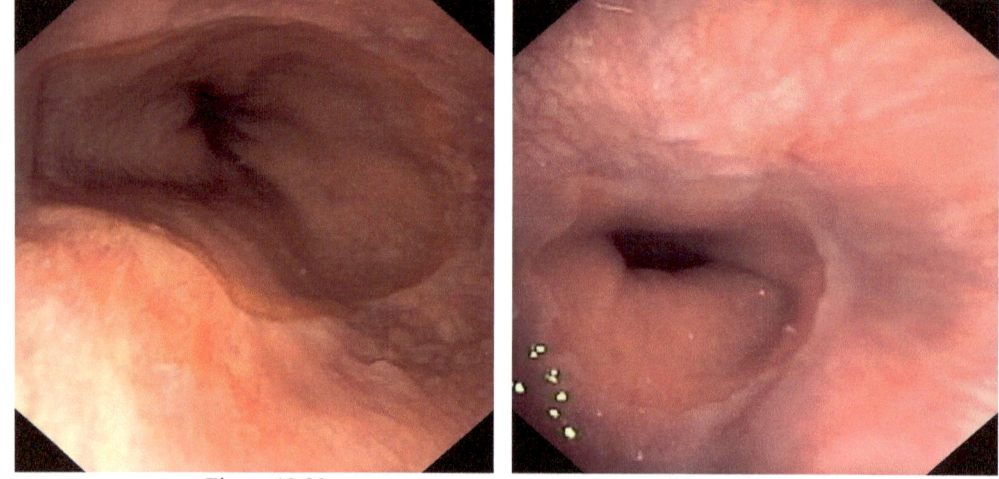

Figure 13.23

Figure 13.24

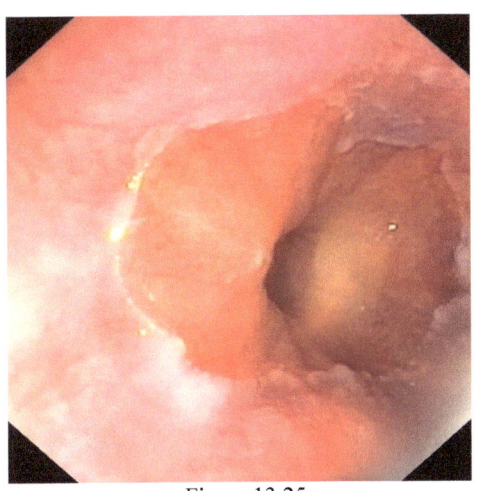

Figure 13.25

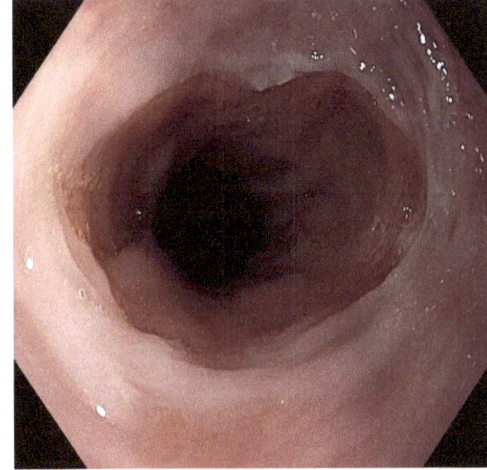

Figure 13.26

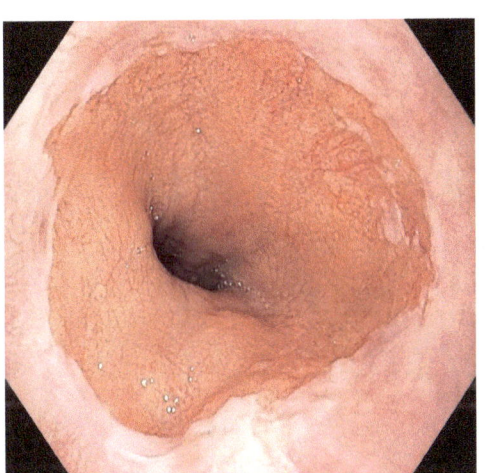

Figure 13.27

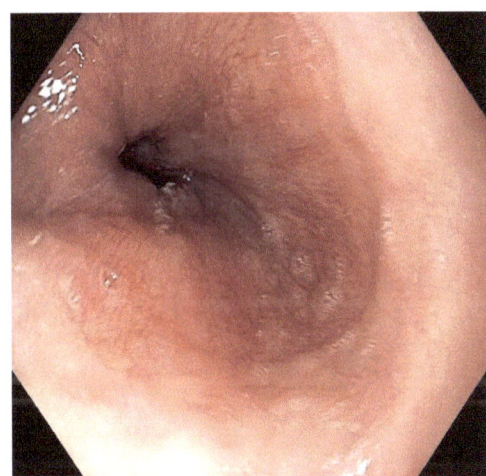

Figure 13.28

Jagged Z-line

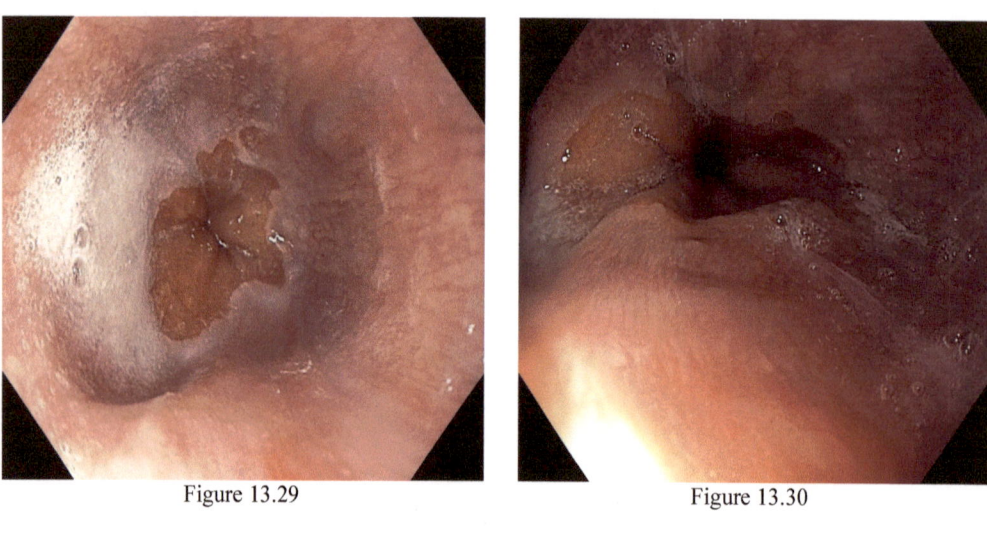

Figure 13.29

Figure 13.30

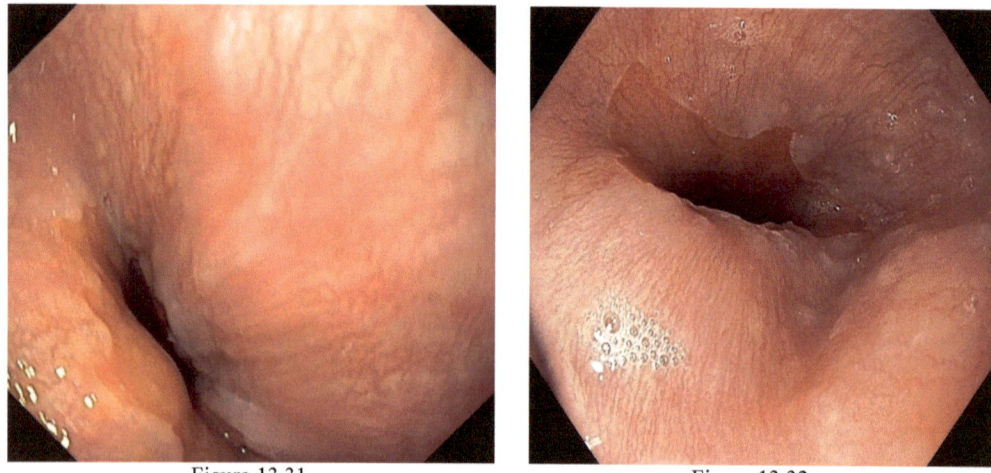

Figure 13.31

Figure 13.32

Flame-shaped Z-line

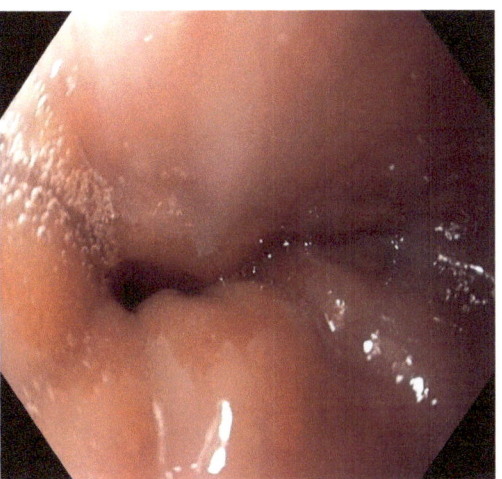
Figure 13.33

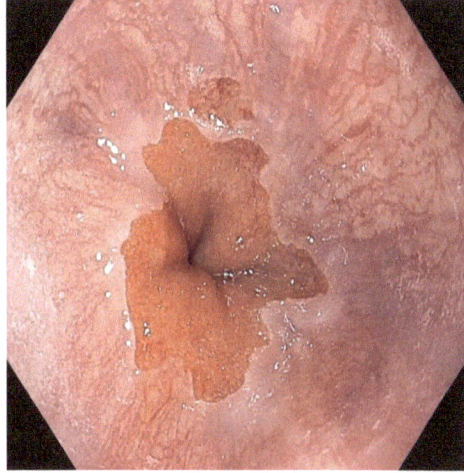
Figure 13.34

Islands of gastric mucosa surrounded by oesophageal mucosa

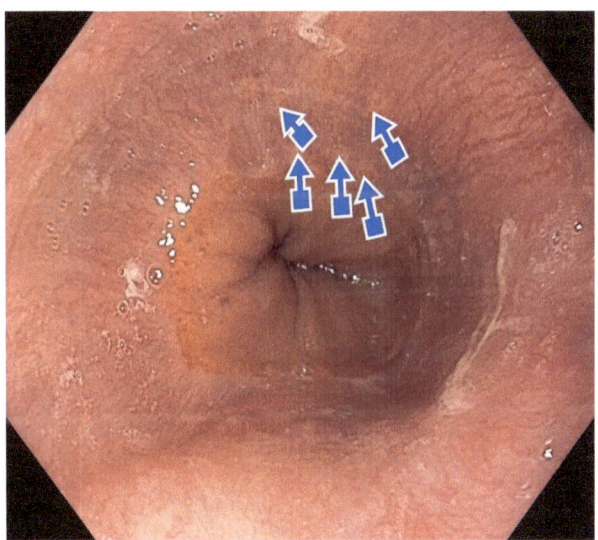
Figure 13.35
The arrows point to islands of gastric mucosa

OESOPHAGEAL ABNORMALITIES

CHAPTER 4

Oesophagitis

This refers to inflammatory changes which may be gross or histological seen in the oesophageal mucosa mostly due to gastroesophageal reflux. The endoscopic pictures include erythema, erosions or ulcerations. Many classification schemes have been proposed to grade oesophagitis, but the most widely used grading system is the Los Angeles System which grades oesophagitis as follows:

Grade A – One (or more) mucosal breaks ≤ 5 mm in length that do not extend between the tops of two mucosal folds

Grade B – One (or more) mucosal breaks > 5 mm in length that do not extend between the tops of two mucosal folds

Grade C – One (or more) mucosal breaks that are continuous between the tops of two or more mucosal folds but involve < 75% of the oesophageal circumference

Grade D – One (or more) mucosal breaks that involve ≥ 75% of the oesophageal circumference

Figures 4.1 and 4.2 are examples of Grade B Oesophagitis. The arrows point to mucosal erosions which are > 5mm in length and do not extend between the tops of two mucosal folds.

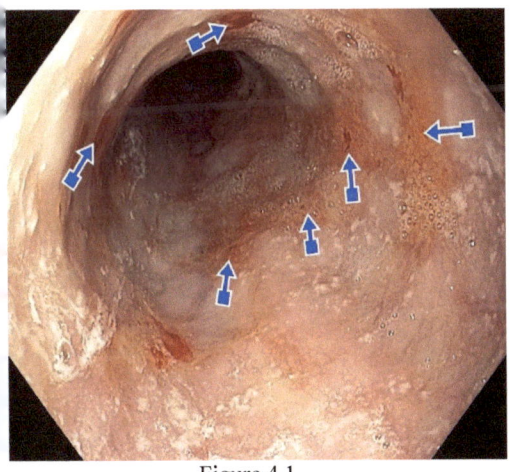 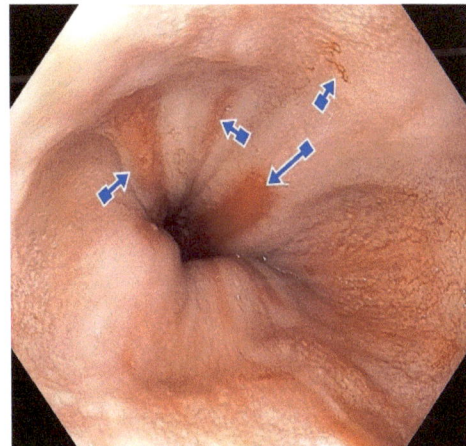

Figure 4.1　　　　　　　　　　　　　　　Figure 4.2

Figures 4.3 is an example of Grade C Oesophagitis. The arrows point to the erosions.

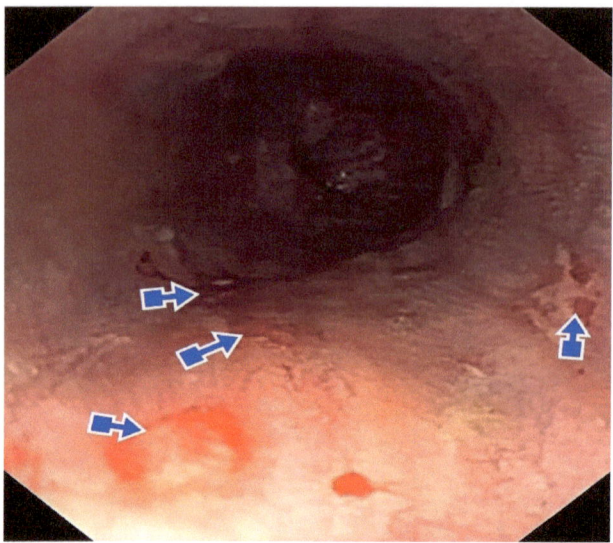

Figure 4.3

Figures 4.4 and 4.5 are examples of Grade D Oesophagitis. The erosions, shown by arrows involve more that 75% of the oesophageal circumference.

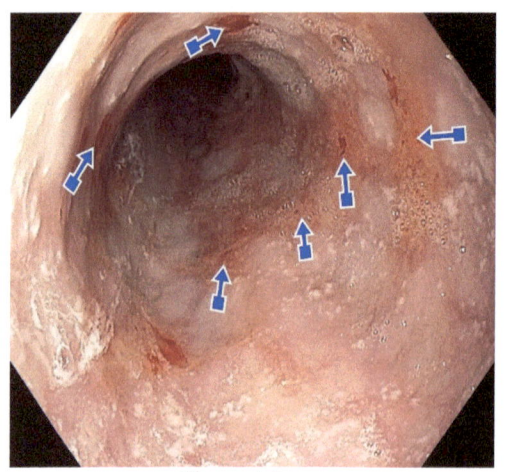 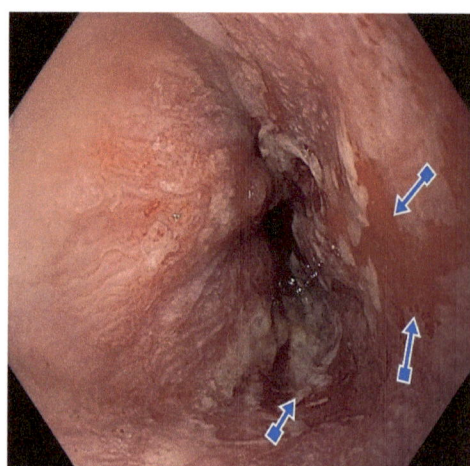

Figure 4.4   Figure 4.5

Oesophageal Ulcers

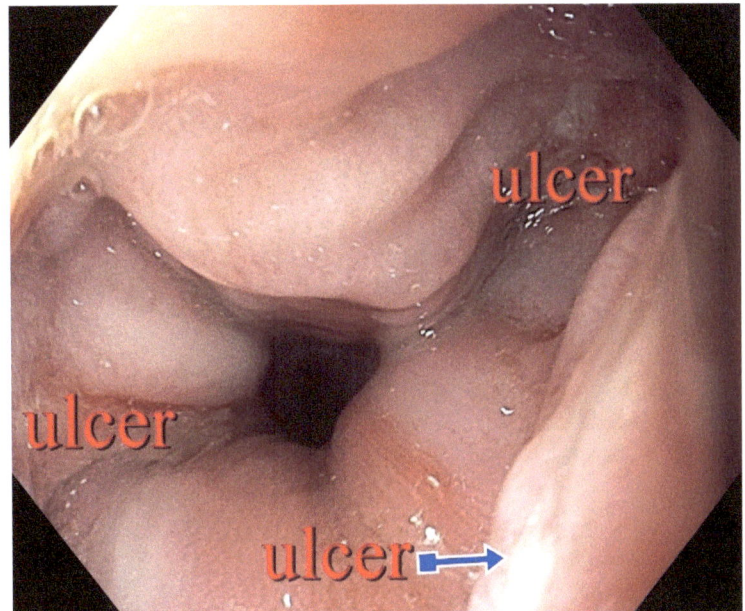

Figure 4.6

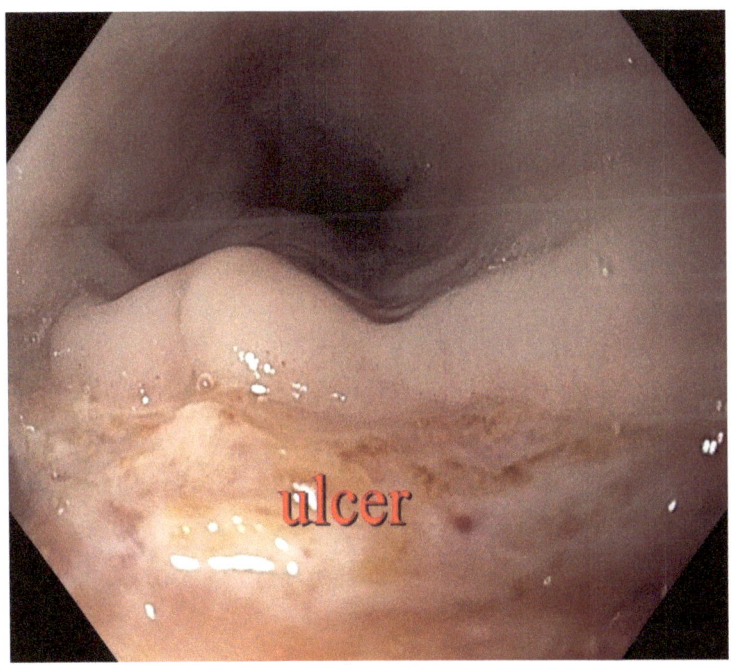

Figure 4.7

Hiatus Hernia

Hernia occurs when an organ or structure protrudes into a pouch or opening. Hiatus hernia occurs when the stomach protrudes through the diaphragmatic hiatus and it is of 3 types:
- Sliding hiatus hernia
- Paraoesophageal hiatus hernia
- Mixed type

Sliding Hiatus Hernia

This is when the gastroesophageal junction (GEJ) and some parts of the stomach move above the diaphragm. In this case, the gastric axis orientation is not disrupted. Although, the aetiology of this condition is not known, it may be due to age-associated weakening of the phrenoesophageal membrane. This may be so because, the incidence of sliding hiatus hernia has been found to increase with advancing age. The phrenoesophageal membrane attaches the GEJ to the diaphragm.

Paraoesophageal Hiatus Hernia

This is when there is protrusion of the stomach through the oesophageal hiatus by the side of the oesophagus. In this case, the position of the GEJ remains at the level of the diaphragm.

However, in most cases of paraoesophageal hernia, a sliding component may be present. This is called *Mixed Hiatus Hernia.*

Occasionally, ulcers may be found in the herniated stomach in hiatus hernia. These ulcers are called Cameron ulcers.

Sliding Hiatus Hernia on Direct View (Figures 4.8 – 4.10)

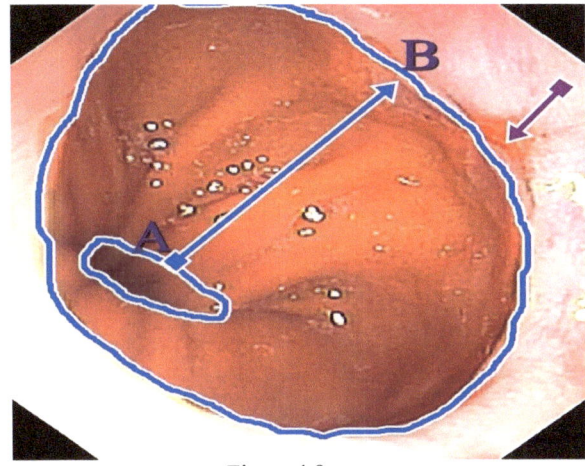

Figure 4.8

Figure 4.8 demonstrates what happens in sliding hiatus hernia. Here, the gastroesophageal junction had shifted from point A, where the diaphragm is to another point B as shown by the BLUE ARROW. The PURPLE ARROW points to Cameron ulcer.

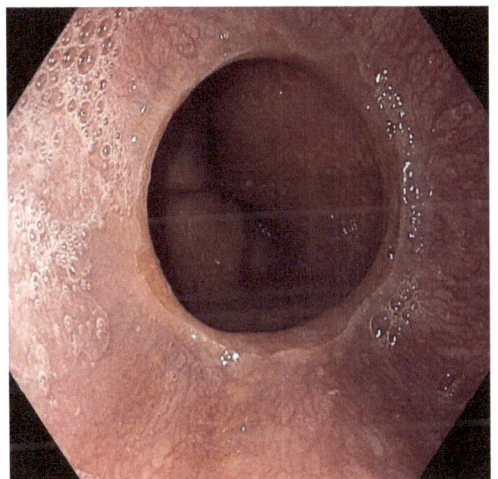   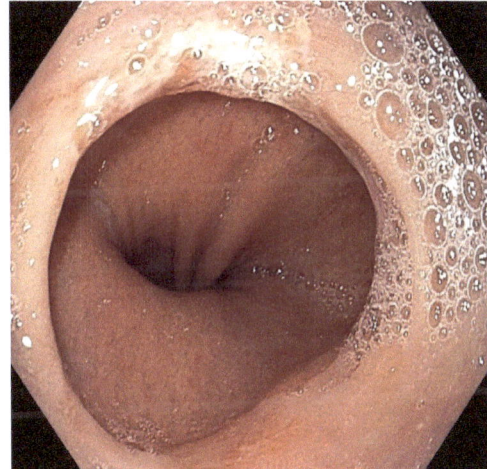

Figure 4.9   Figure 4.10

Sliding Hiatus Hernia during Retroflexion of the Endoscope

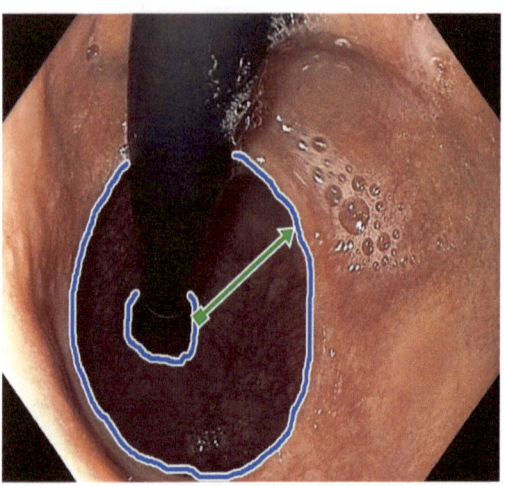
Figure 4.11

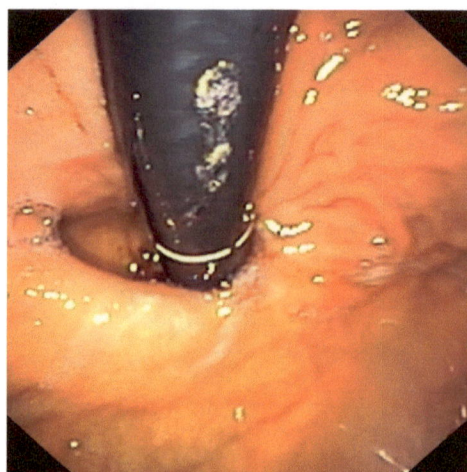
Figure 4.12

In figure 4.11, the green arrow showed the shifted gastroesophageal junction and part of the stomach. This can actually be measured using the scale on the scope. In this particular instance, it is about 3 cm.

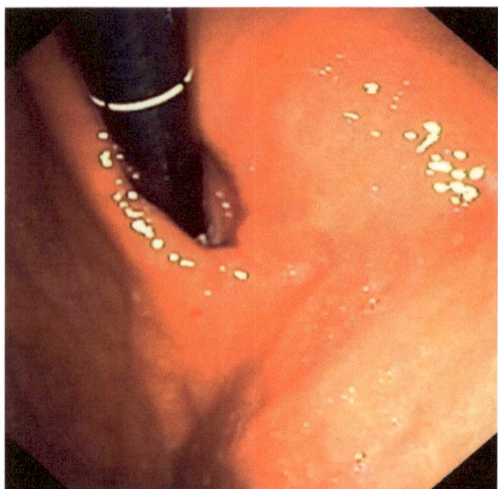
Figure 4.13

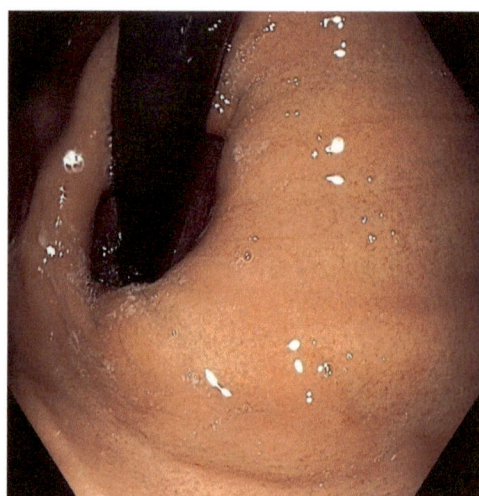
Figure 4.14

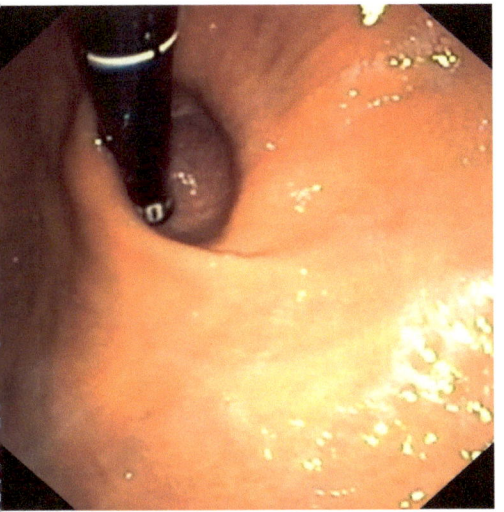 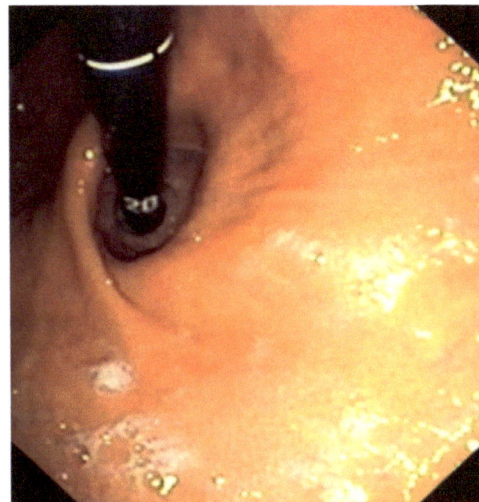

Figure 4.15   Figure 4.16

Barrett's Oesophagus

This is an acquired disorder secondary to severe injury of the oesophageal mucosa. At endoscopy, there is proximal displacement of the squamocolumnar junction above the gastroesophageal junction (GEJ). This is confirmed by the detection of intestinal metaplasia on oesophageal biopsy. Barrett's oesophagus is a premalignant condition, which has been found to have association with oesophageal adenocarcinoma. Gastroesophageal reflux disease (GERD) is a predisposing condition to Barrett's oesophagus. About 6-12% of patients with GERD have been reported to have Barrett's. Based on the length of the displaced squamocolumnar junction, there are 2 types:
- Short-segment Barrett's, when it is < 3 cm in length
- Long-segment Barrett's, when it is ≥ 3 cm in length

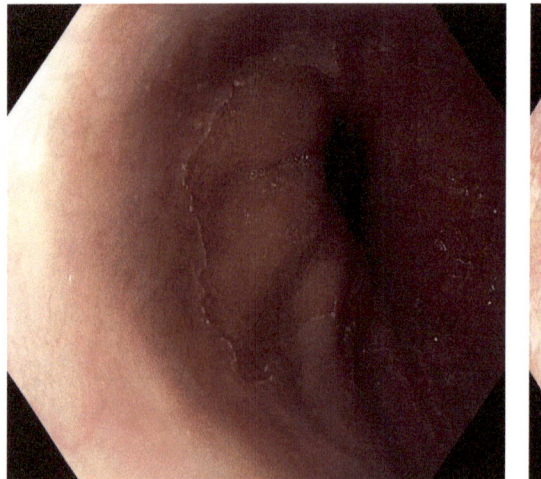
Figure 4.17

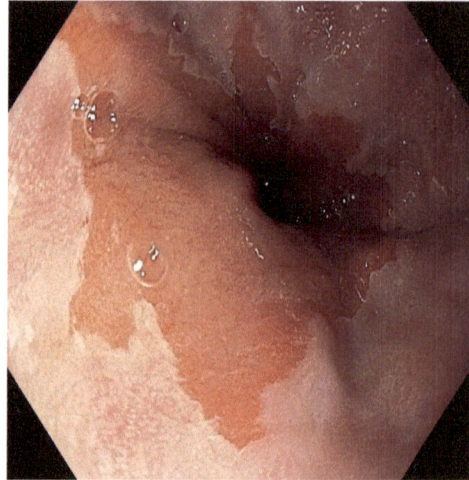
Figure 4.18

Oesophageal Candidiasis

The main cause of oesophageal candidiasis is *Candida albicans,* which is found in normal oral flora. Other human fungal commensal organisms are *Candida glabrata, C. krusei, C. parapsilosis, C. tropicalis.* Two stages are involved in the mucosal infection by *C. albicans:* First is colonization, which is characterized by superficial adherence and proliferation, the second step is invasion of the epithelium and this requires a defective cellular immunity. The infection is characterized by whitish adherent plaques on the mucosa. When these plaques are removed, a raw and friable surface is exposed.

The most significant risk factor for oesophageal candidiasis is HIV infection. Other risk factors are diabetes mellitus, malignancies, alcoholism, adrenal dysfunction, progressive systemic sclerosis, achalasia, steroid and immunosuppressive therapy, and hypochlorhydria.

Oesophageal candidiasis is mostly asymptomatic, but patients sometimes complain of dysphagia and/or odynophagia.

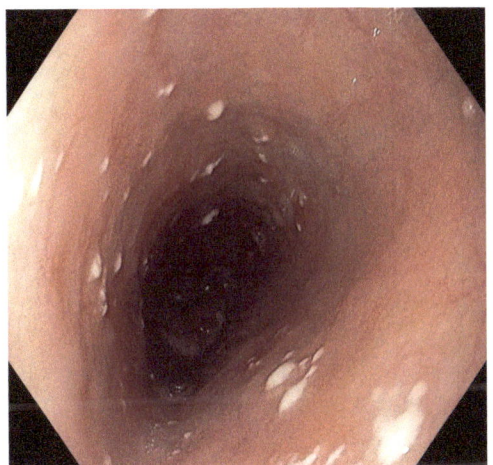

Figure 4.19

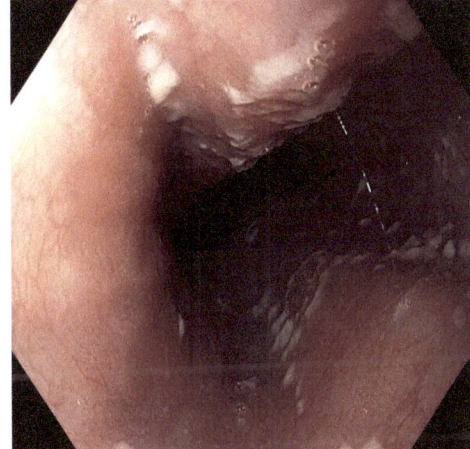

Figure 4.20

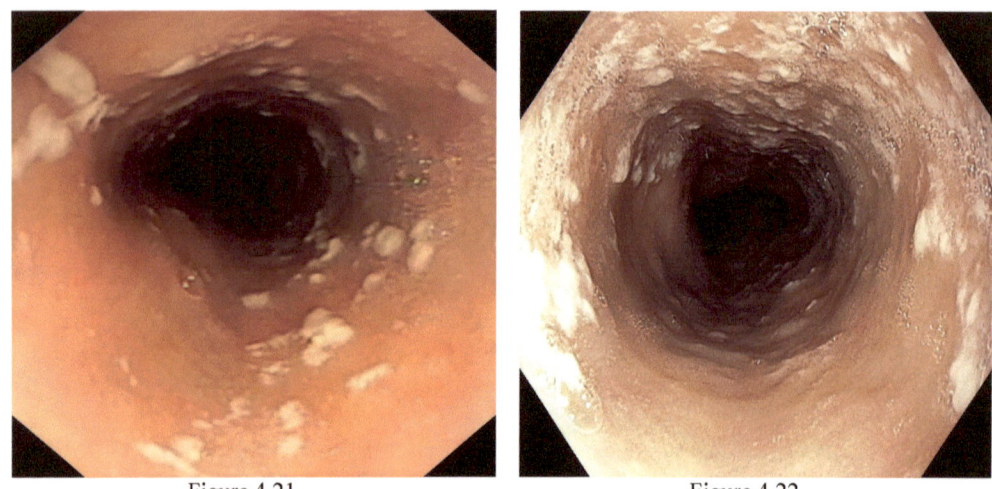

| Figure 4.21 | Figure 4.22 |

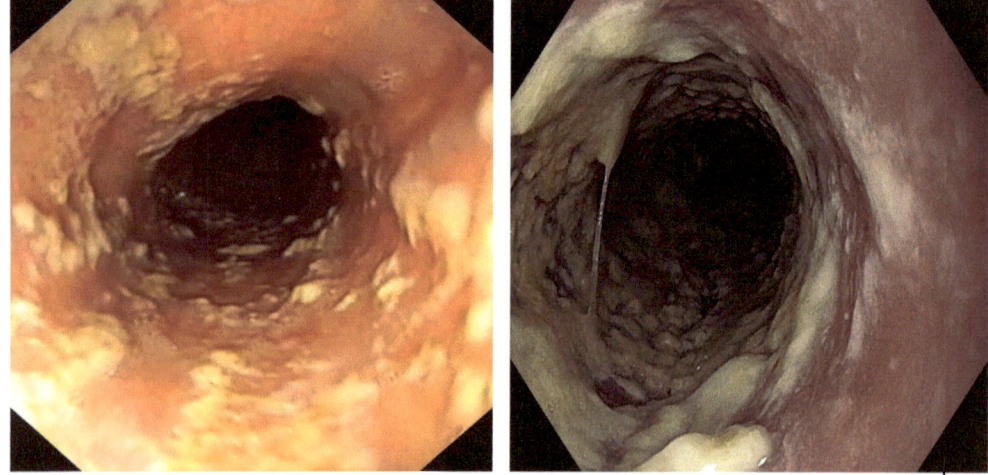

| Figure 4.23 | Figure 4.24 |

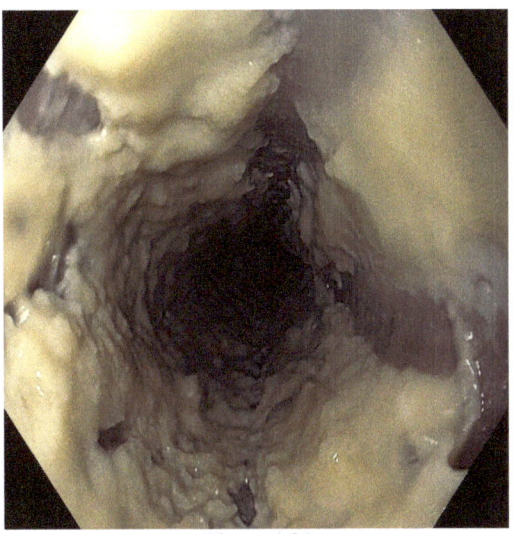 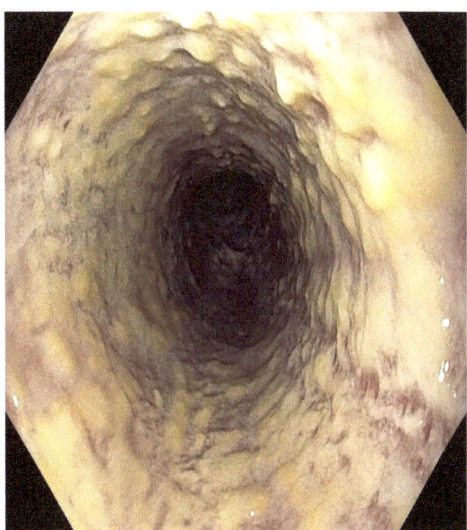

Figure 4.25   Figure 4.26

Oesophageal Varices

Varices are natural shunts or collaterals between the portal and the systemic circulations that result from portal hypertension. Portal hypertension is a major complication of liver cirrhosis and is said to occur when the portal venous pressure is greater than 5 mm Hg. Varices occur in areas where both the systemic venous and the portal venous systems appose. Such areas are gastroesophageal junction (GEJ), stomach, anorectum, around the umbilicus, ovaries, retroperitoneal space, bare area of the liver.

About half of patients with liver cirrhosis develop oesophageal varices, and about 20% of these patients have large varices. Upper gastrointestinal endoscopy can easily diagnose oesophageal varices, and they are mostly located in the distal oesophagus. There are several classifications for grading varices, however, the size of the varices can simply be graded as follows:
- Small varices : 1-3 mm in diameter
- Medium varices: 3-6 mm in diameter
- Large varices : >6 mm in diameter

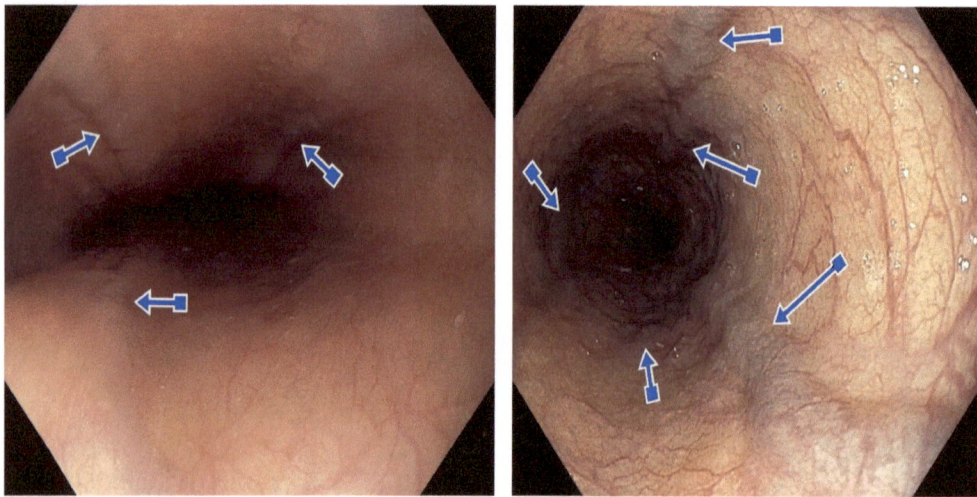

Figure 4.27　　　　　　　　　　　　Figure 4.28

In figures 4.27 and 4.28, the arrows point to the varices. In figure 4.27, they are 'WHITE', whereas in figure 4.28, they are 'BLUE'

Also, on the varices, there are features that can be identified which are signs of imminent rupture of such varices. These features are called Red Colour Signs. They are 3 types:

- ✓ Red wale markings (Red thin arrows in figures 4.33 & 4.34)
- ✓ Cherry red spots   (Red thick arrows in figures 4.34 & 4.35)
- ✓ Haematocytic spots (Brown thin arrows in figure 4.36)

There are also signs that appear after haemostasis of a bleeding varix. These are called 'plugs', which could be red or white. (Figure 4.30)

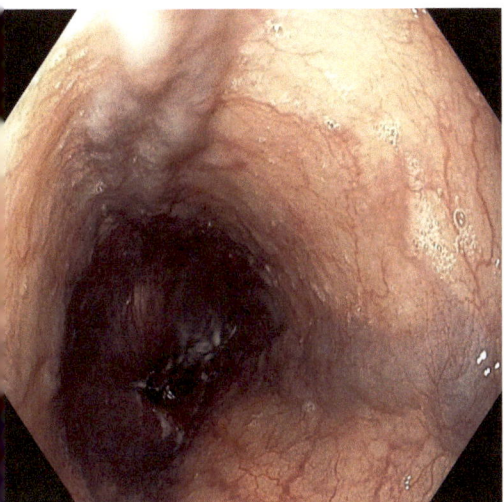
Figure 4.29

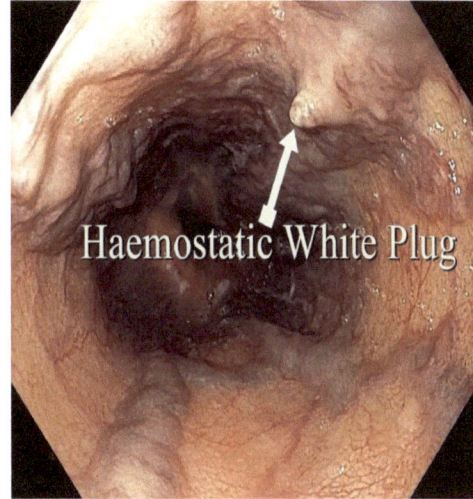
Figure 4.30

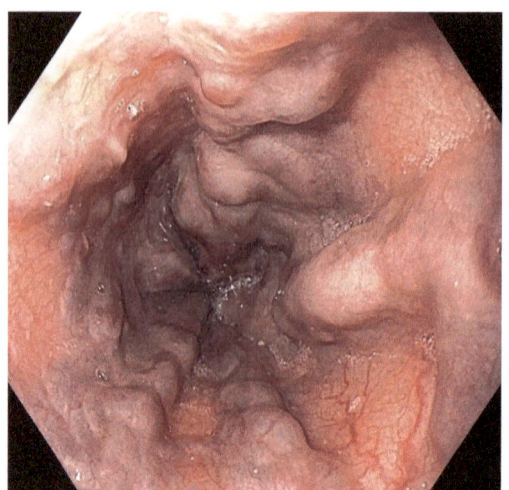

Figure 4.31

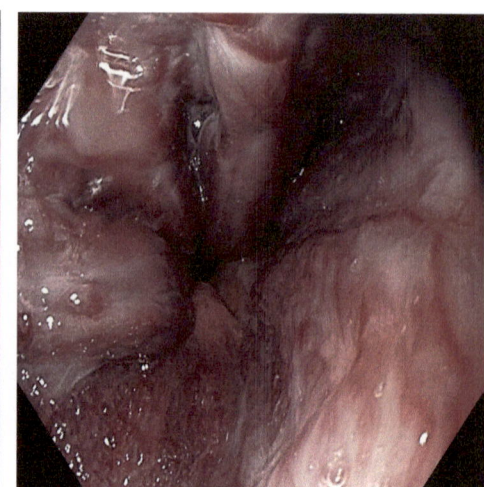

Figure 4.32

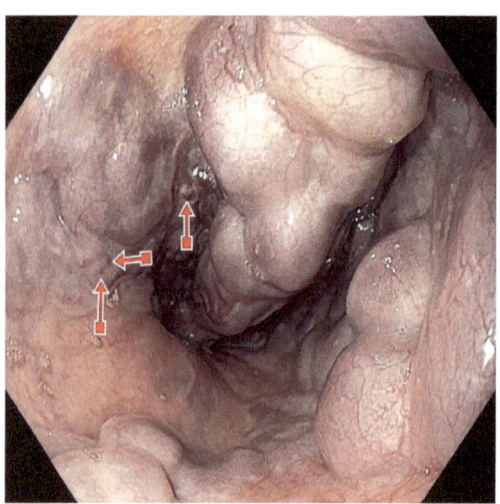

Figure 4.33

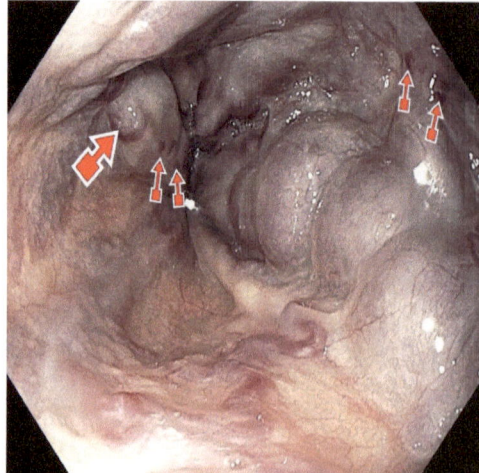

Figure 4.34

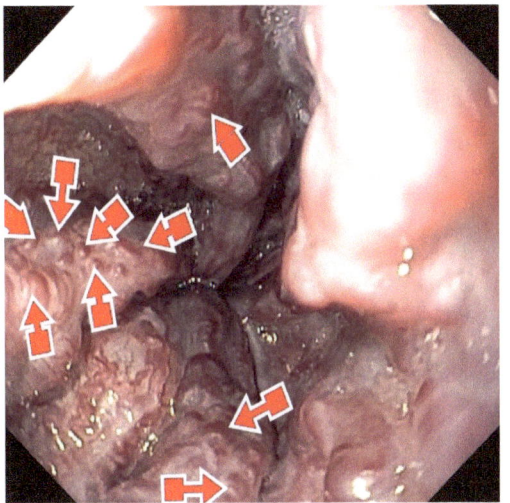
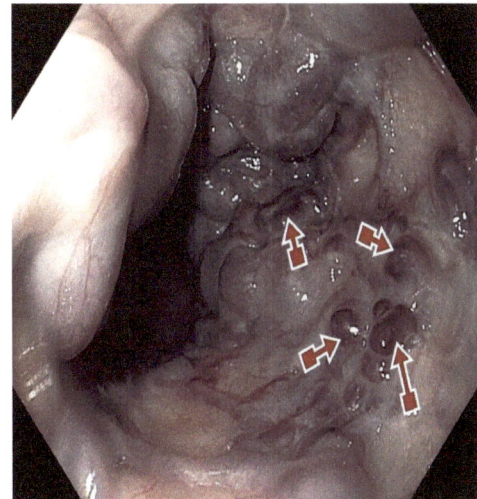

Figure 4.35   Figure 4.36

Variceal Band Ligation/Endoscopic Variceal Ligation (VBL or EVL)

This is a technique that is used to control oesophageal variceal bleeding. It is effective both for primary, as well as for secondary prophylaxis of variceal haemorrhage. During the procedure, a plastic cylinder which has been preloaded with rubber bands is inserted into the tip of a forward viewing endoscope, which is then introduced into the oesophagus. The tip of the cylinder is brought close to a varix, which is then suctioned effectively into the cylinder until a red out is seen. Thereafter, a rubber band is deployed around the base of the varix with the help of a trigger device already placed at the tip of the biopsy channel of the endoscope. Usually, in one session up to 5-8 bands can be deployed circumferentially. This can be repeated every 4-6 weeks until all the varices have been banded.

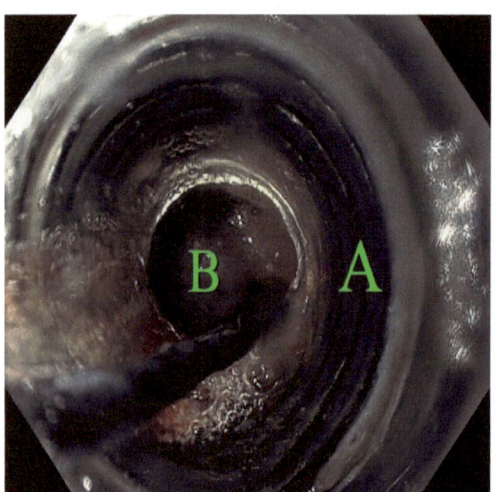
Figure 4.37

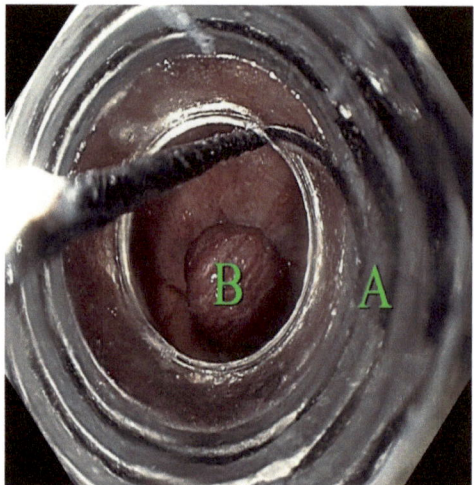
Figure 4.38

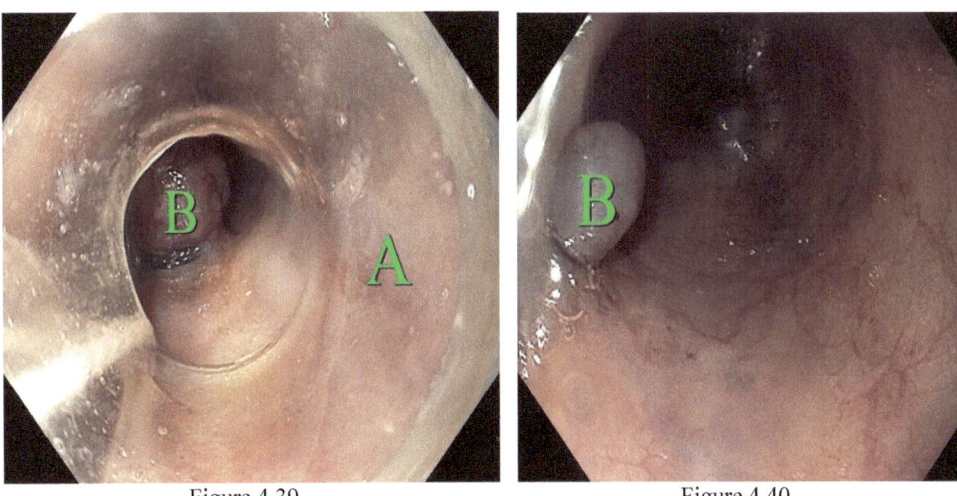

Figure 4.39　　　　　　　　　　　　Figure 4.40
In figures 4.37- 4.40: A- shooter barrel with the bands, B- varix with band at the base

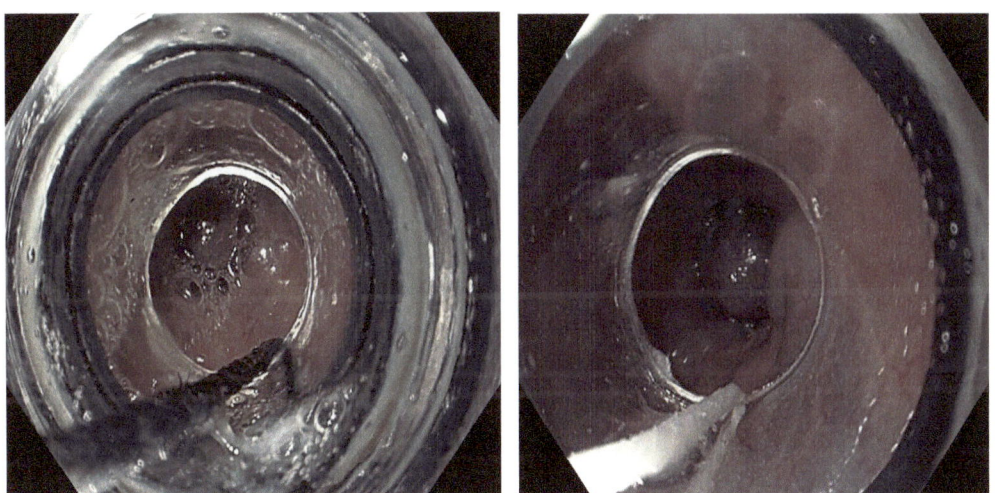

Figure 4.41　　　　　　　　　　　　Figure 4.42

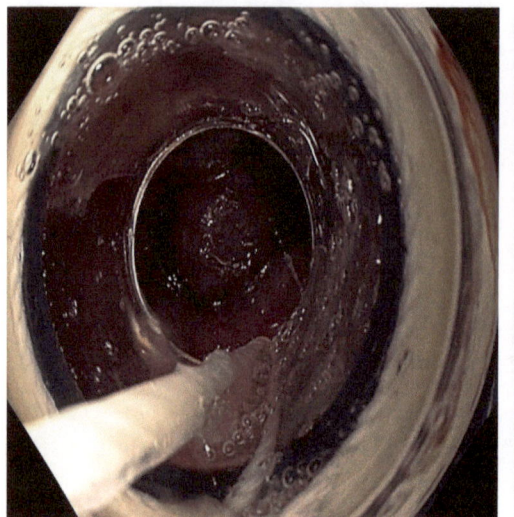 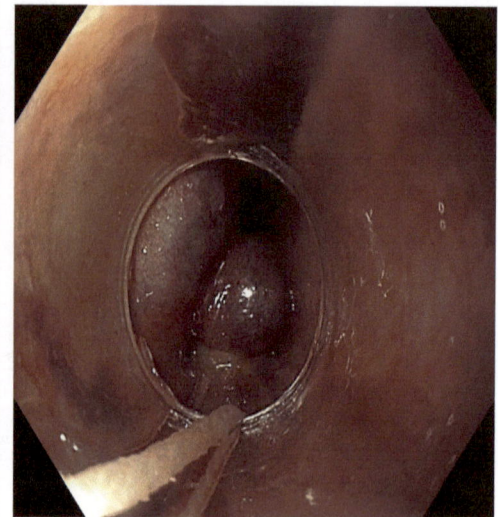

Figure 4.43 Figure 4.44

Oesophageal Carcinoma

Oesophageal carcinoma is a highly lethal condition and the 5th cause of cancer death globally. Most patients present late when the disease is already advanced. The subtypes are:
- Squamous cell carcinoma (SCCA)
- Adenocarcinoma (AdenoCA)
- Verrucous carcinoma
- Small cell carcinoma

The most common type in the world is the SCCA, while in Europe and the USA there has been an increase in the incidence of AdenoCA. SCCA is seen more commonly in blacks, while AdenoCA affects white men more. Most AdenoCA arises from intestinal metaplasia (Barrett's oesophagus) and as such, one risk factor for oesophageal AdenoCA is symptomatic GERD.

The accuracy of endoscopy when combined with biopsy and cytology in diagnosing upper gastrointestinal cancers is about 100%. It has a higher sensitivity and specificity compared to double-contrast barium studies.

Early oesophageal cancer can be in form of minor mucosal irregularities, areas of depression or erythema; sometimes ulcerated or raised areas. Advanced lesions can be polypoid or ulcerated and are usually obvious.

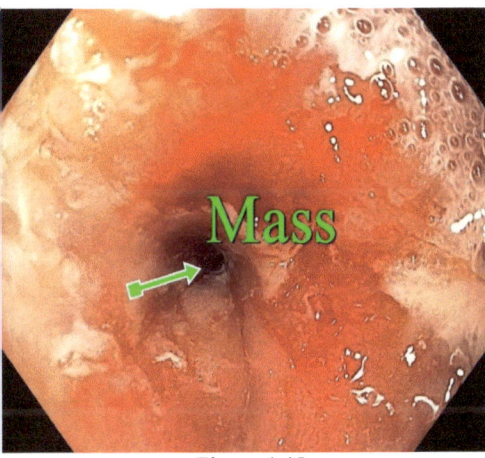
Figure 4.45

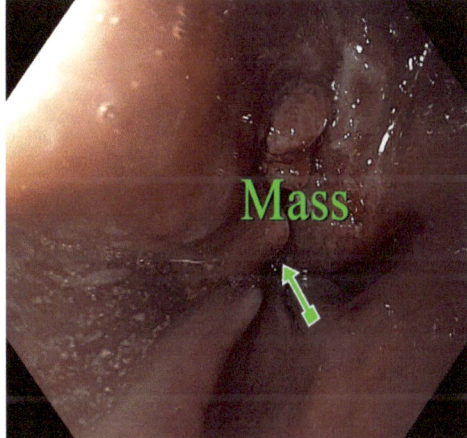
Figure 4.46

In these pictures, the oesophageal mass is circumferential, thereby causing complete obstruction of the lumen. The arrow points to what is left of the lumen, which is like pin-hole.

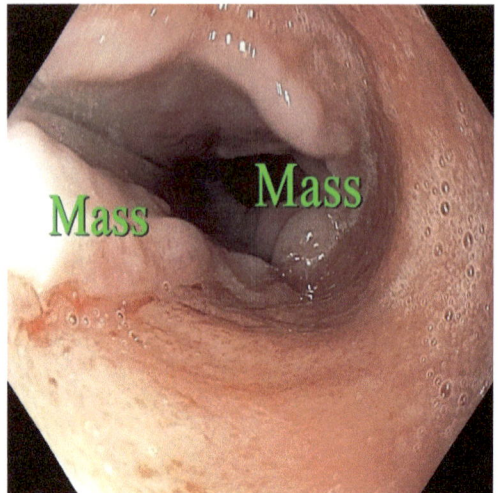

Figure 4.47

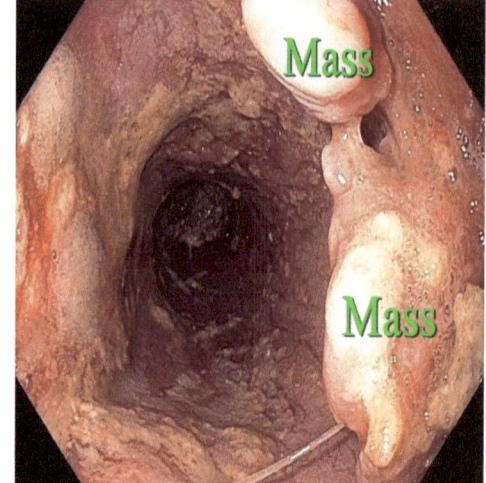

Figure 4.48

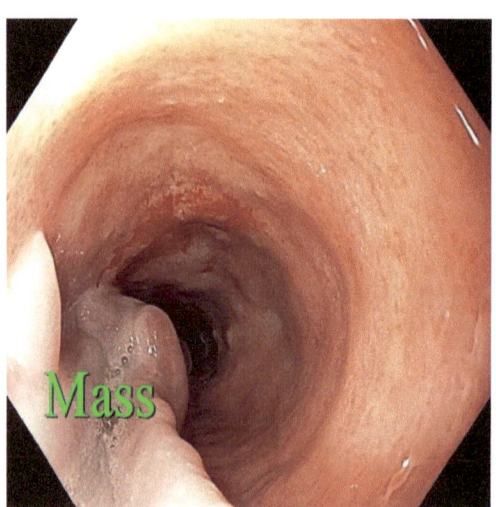

Figure 4.49

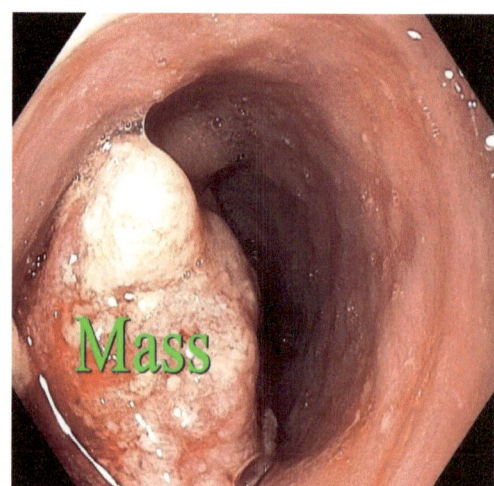

Figure 4.50

Oesophageal Foreign Bodies

In adults, accidental ingestion of foreign bodies occur in certain groups of people, like the very elderly, demented or intoxicated individuals. Psychiatric patients, as well as prisoners tend to ingest foreign bodies intentionally. The most common risk factors that encourage accidental ingestion of foreign bodies are dentures or dental work which may cause impaired tactile sensation when swallowing. Food impaction in the oesophagus is more common than other foreign body ingestion.

Some oesophageal abnormalities that predispose to food impaction are peptic strictures, Schatzki's rings, extrinsic compression, webs, achalasia, diffuse oesophageal spasm and nutcracker oesophagus. There are four areas of physical narrowing in the oesophagus where foreign bodies may lodge. These are:
- Upper oesophageal sphincter
- Level of the aortic arch
- Level of the crossing of the main bronchus
- Gastroesophageal junction and the lower oesophageal sphincter

The most accurate diagnostic method when foreign body ingestion is suspected is endoscopy. It also helps to diagnose the underlying predisposing pathology. It is also useful in assessing mucosal damage from the ingested foreign body, as well as for treatment or extraction of some foreign bodies.

Predisposing Conditions to Oesophageal Foreign Body Impaction

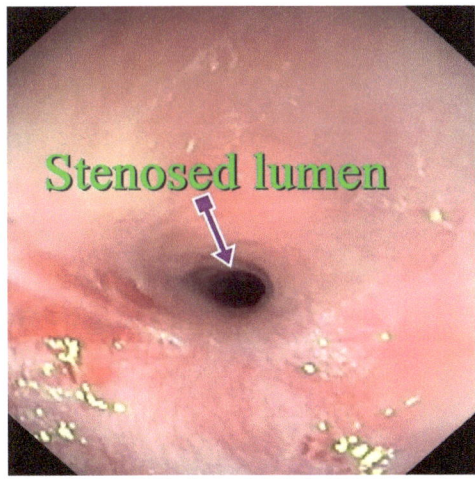 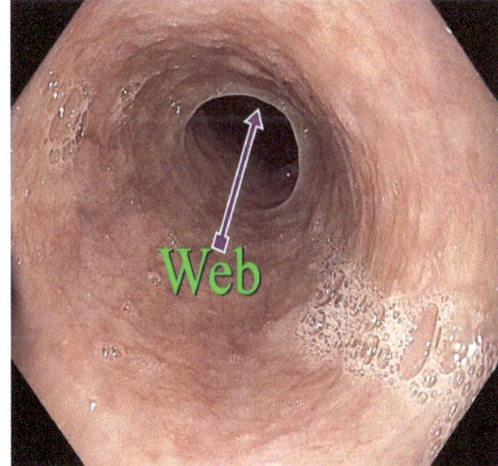

Figure 4.51: Oesophageal stricture   Figure 4.52: Oesophageal web

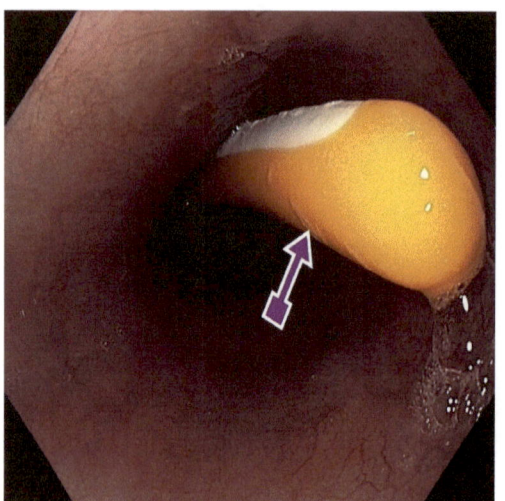

Figure 4.53
Swallowed toothbrush in the oesophagus

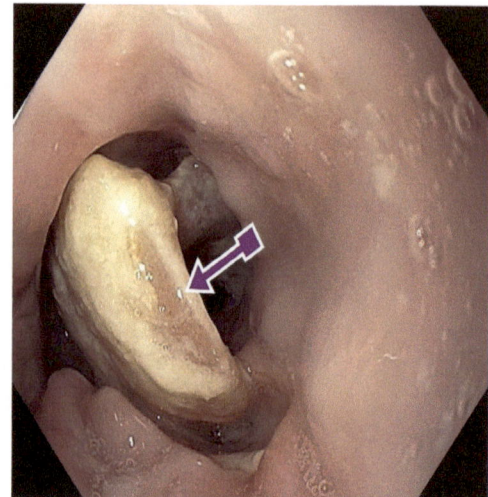

Figure 4.54
Swallowed denture in the oesophagus

Other Oesophageal Abnormalities

(I) Achalasia

In this condition, there is incomplete relaxation, as well as hypertonicity of the lower oesophageal sphincter (LES). There is progressive worsening of LES dysfunction, followed by loss of oesophageal peristalsis, oesophageal dilatation and eventual oesophageal failure.

Symptoms include dysphagia to both solids and liquids, chest pain, and regurgitation.
Endoscopic findings include:
- A tight gastroesophageal junction/lower oesophageal sphincter area (Figure 4.55)
- Oesophageal dilatation (Figure 4.56)
- Presence of pooled saliva or retained food in the oesophagus (Figure 4.57)
- May be normal, especially in early cases

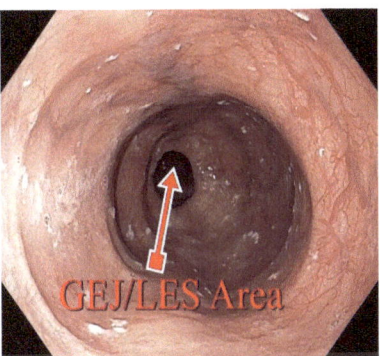 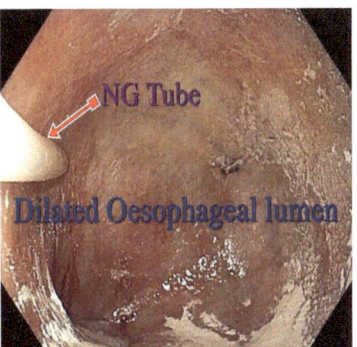

Figure 4.55   Figure 4.56

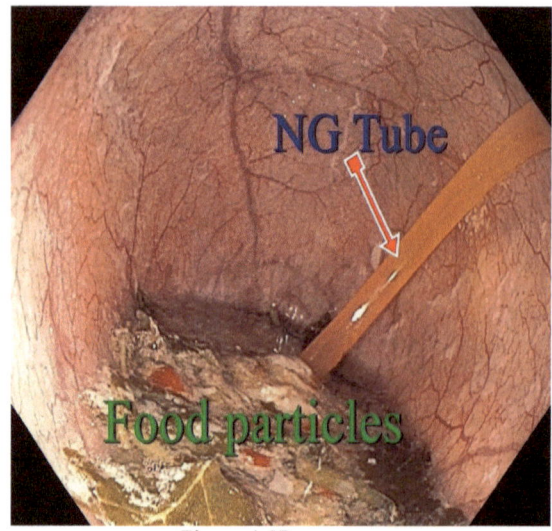

Figure 4.57

(II) Oesophageal Angiodysplasia (Figure 4.58)

(III) Oesophageal Polyp (Figure 4.59)

(IV) Oesophageal Diverticulum (Figure 4.60)

(V) Oesophageal Rings (Figure 4.61)

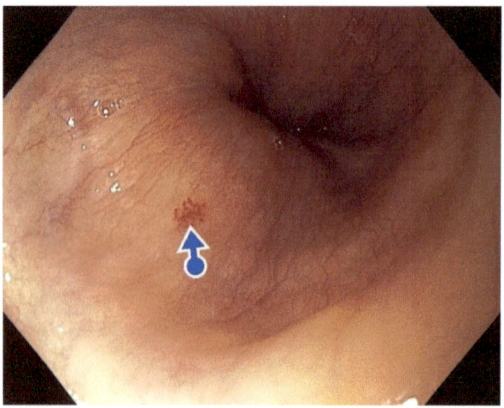

Figure 4.58

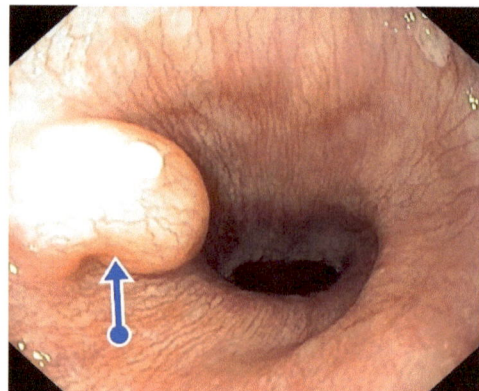

Figure 4.59

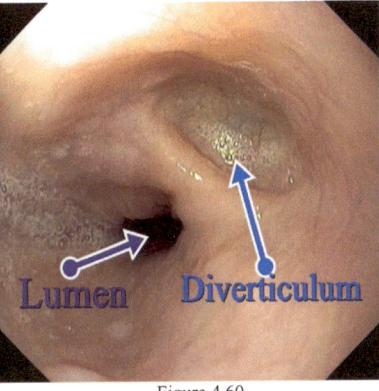

Figure 4.60

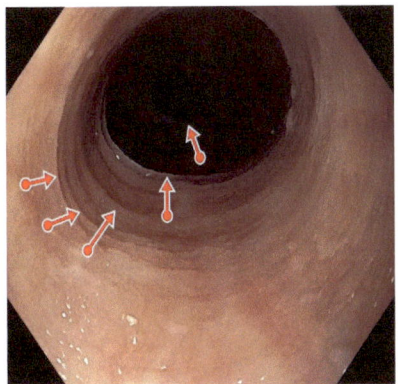

Figure 4.61

STOMACH

50

CHAPTER 5

Normal Stomach

The region that is seen after passing the scope through the gastroesophageal junction/lower oesophageal sphincter is the interior of the stomach.
The various parts of the stomach are:
- Cardia
- Fundus
- Body
- Antrum

Upon entry into the stomach, the first portion that is seen is the junction of the fundus and body where a small quantity of resting juice can be visualized.

Gastric Body (Corpus)

It has the shape of a funnel with tortuous mucosal folds (rugae). With maximal distention of the lumen, the folds tend to straighten out. The gastric mucosa usually appears reddish-orange in colour. If the mucosa becomes atrophic, visible networks of vessels may be present.

With the position of the scope in the body of the stomach, the lesser curvature is to the right, while the greater curvature is to the left. Also, on the left is the anterior gastric wall, while the posterior wall is on the right with patient in the left lateral position.

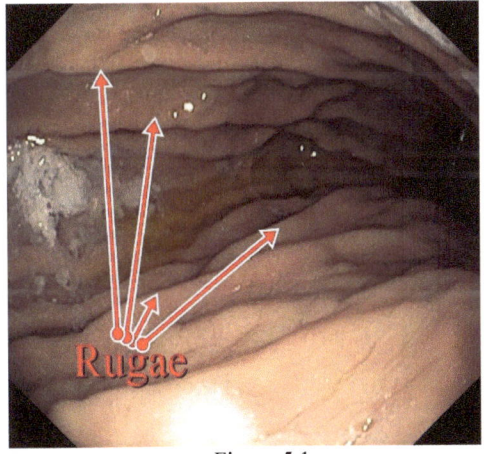
Figure 5.1

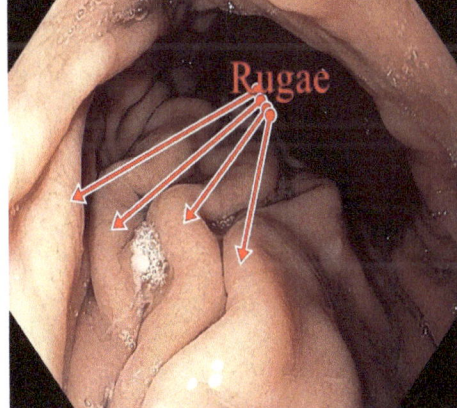
Figure 5.2

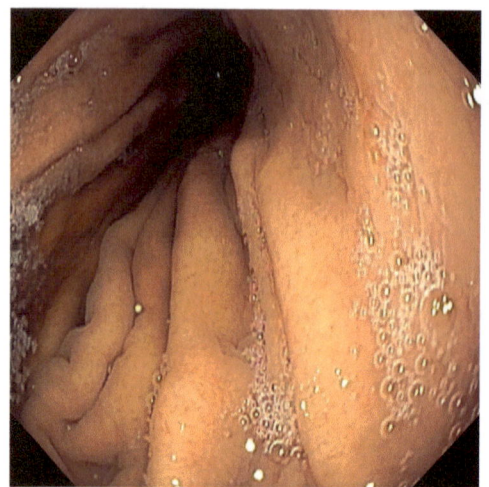

Figure 5.3

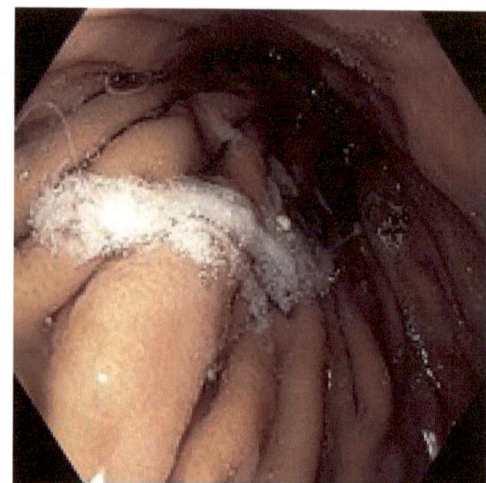

Figure 5.4

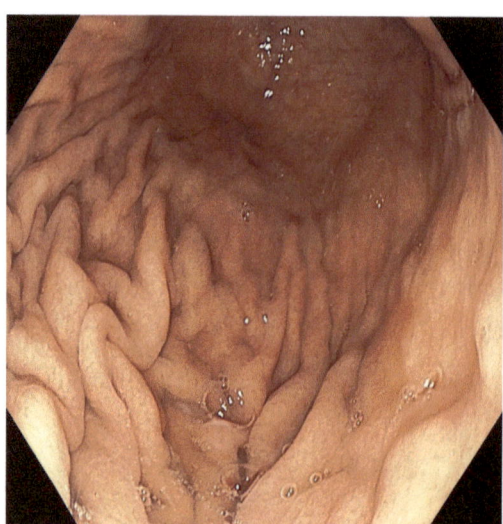

Figure 5.5

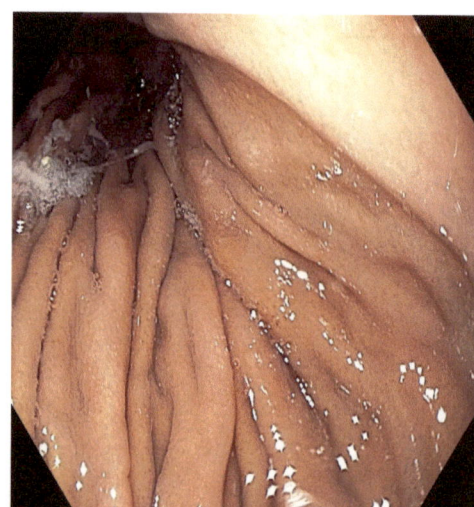

Figure 5.6

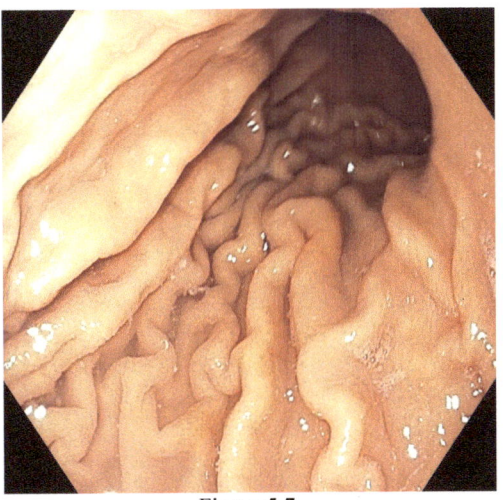

Figure 5.7

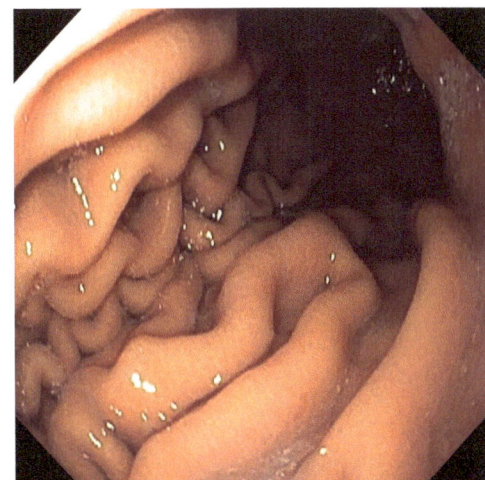

Figure 5.8

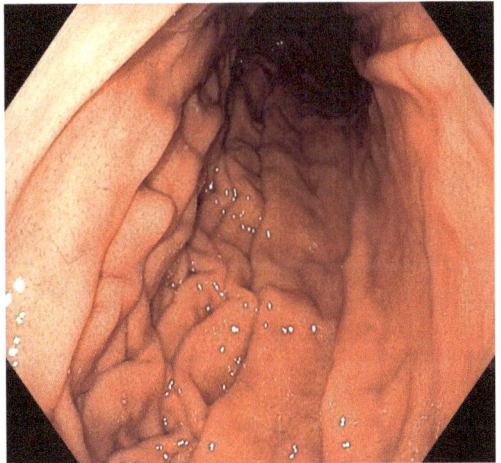

Figure 5.9

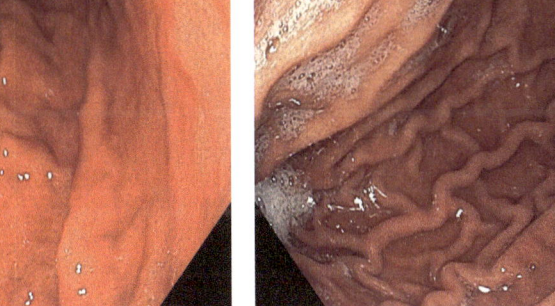

Figure 5.10

Gastric Antrum

As one proceeds from the stomach body(corpus) to the antrum, the gastric folds(rugae) become less prominent and transits to the smooth mucosa of the antrum. In other words, there are no folds in the antrum. However, in some very rare cases, some folds may extend into the antrum.

Incisura angularis marks the end of the body and the beginning of the antrum. The antrum is dome-shaped with the pyloric opening at its tip. It is usual to find folds around the pylorus during contraction. The antrum has smooth mucosa which may be yellowish-gray or reddish-orange in appearance.

Antrum

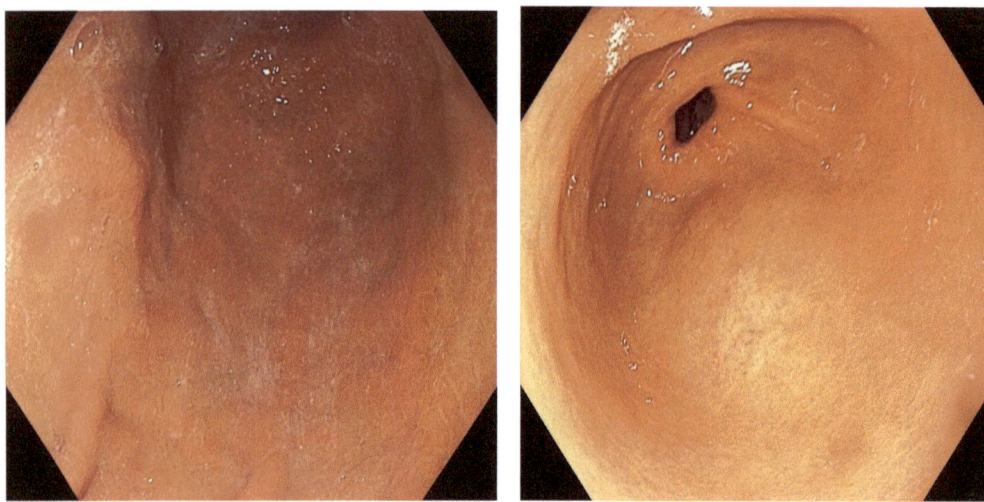

Figure 5.11   Figure 5.12

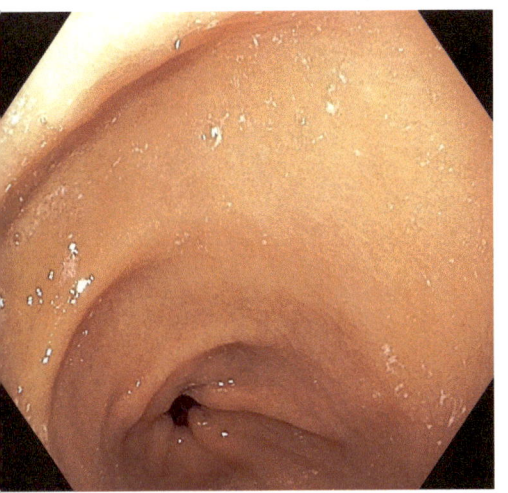

Figure 5.13

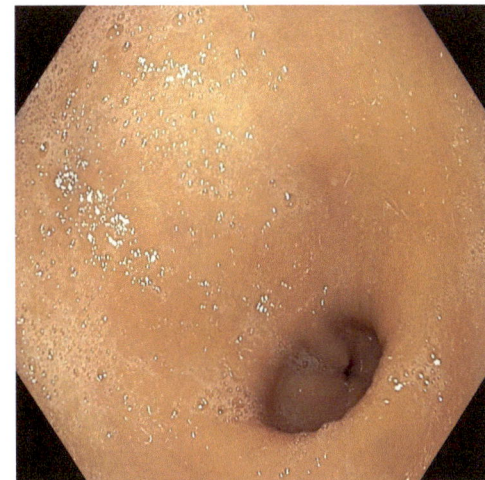

Figure 5.14

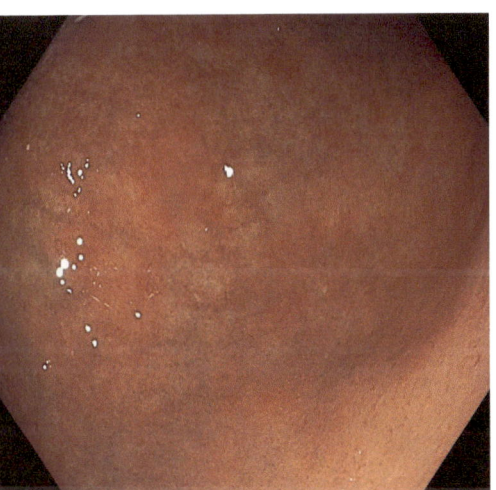

Figure 5.15

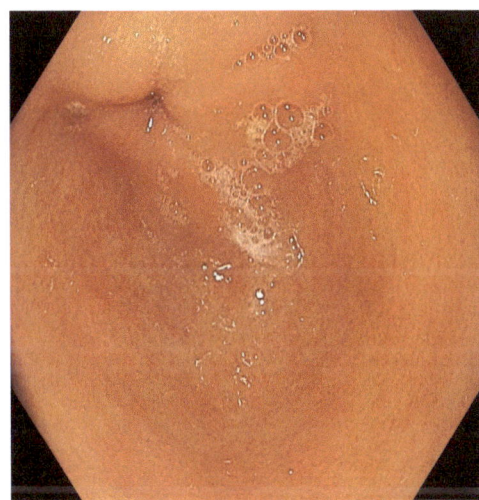

Figure 5.16

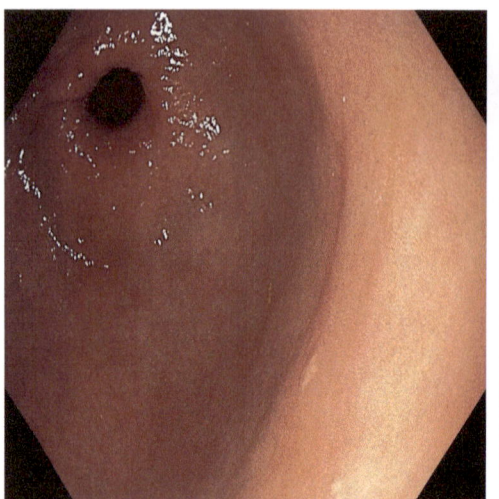

Figure 5.17

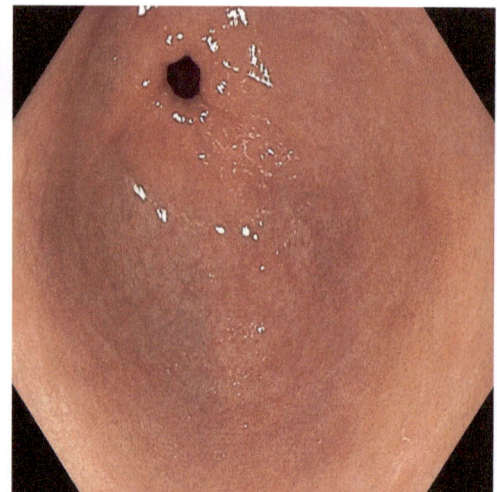

Figure 5.18

Incisura during direct viewing

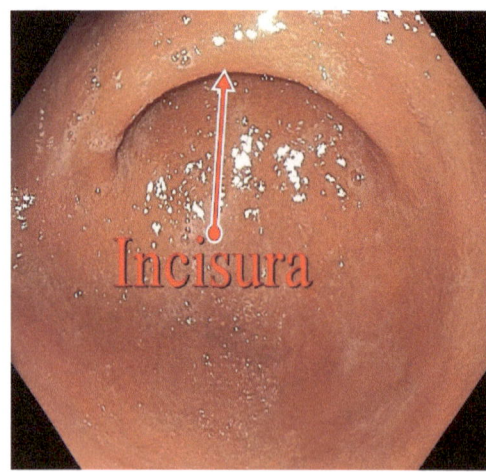

Figure 5.19

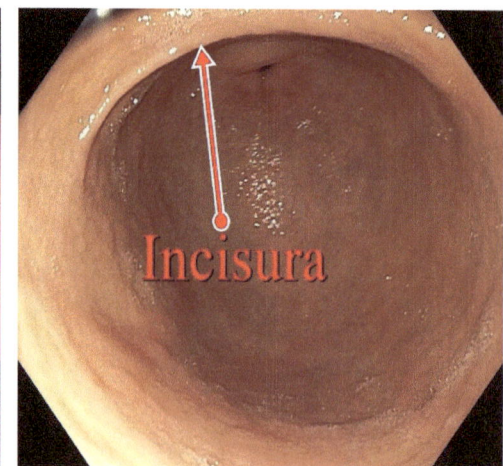

Figure 5.20

Incisura during retroflexion

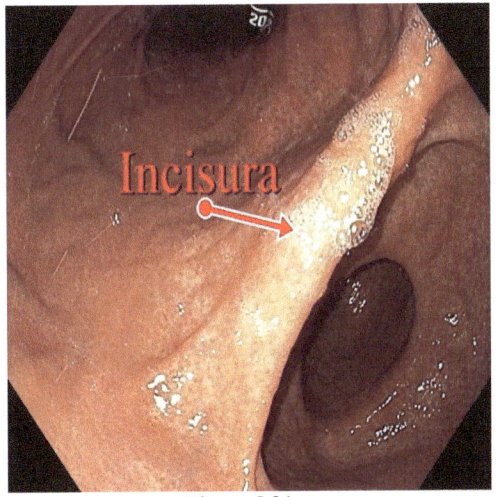

Figure 5.21

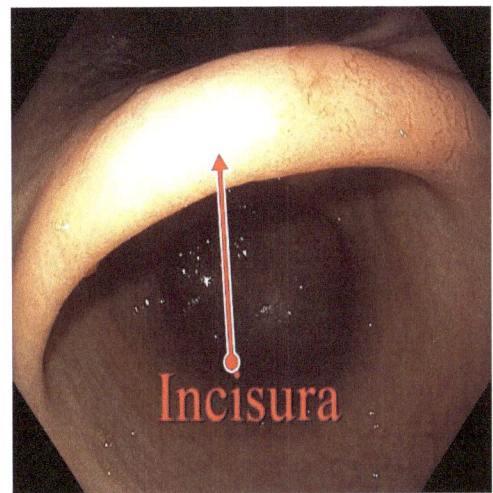

Figure 5.22

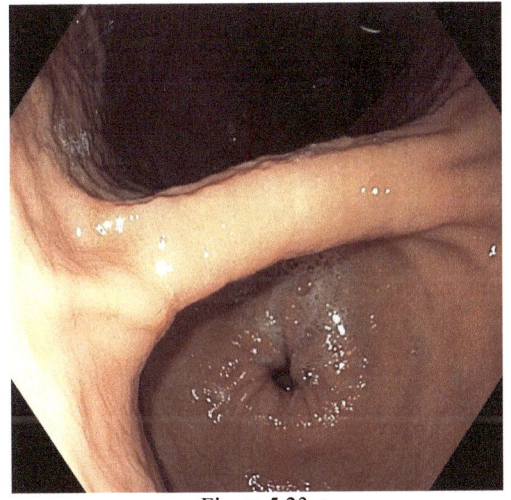

Figure 5.23

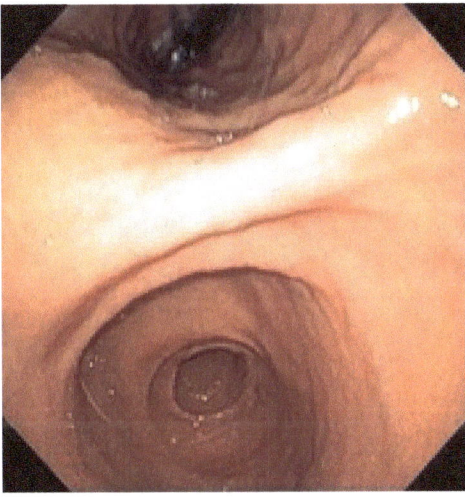

Figure 5.24

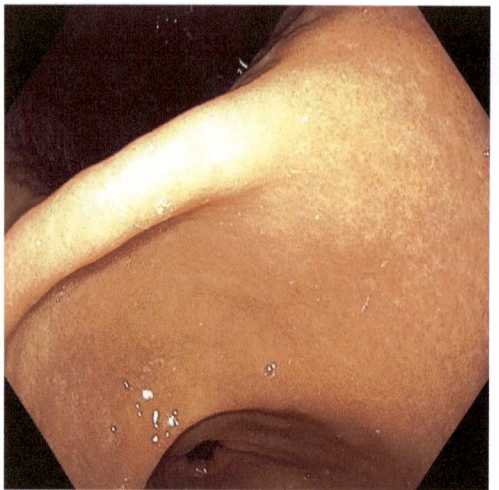
Figure 5.25

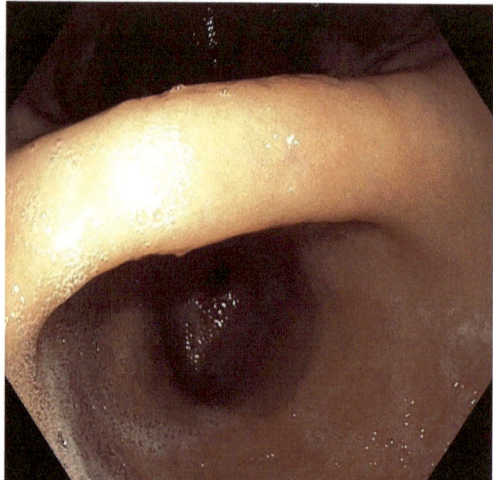
Figure 5.26

Pylorus at different stages of relaxation

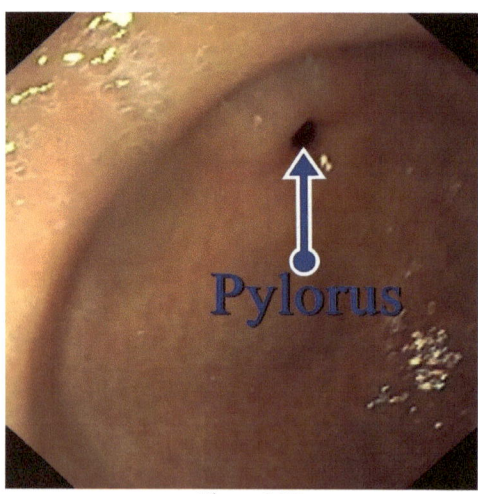
Figure 5.27

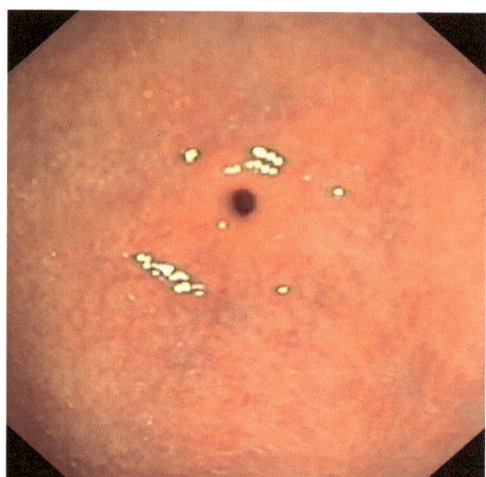
Figure 5.28

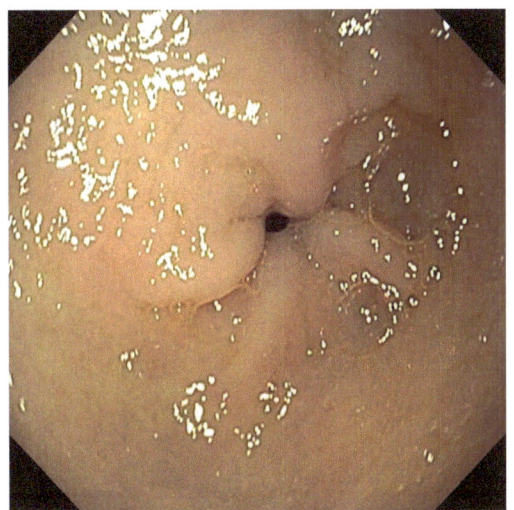

Figure 5.29

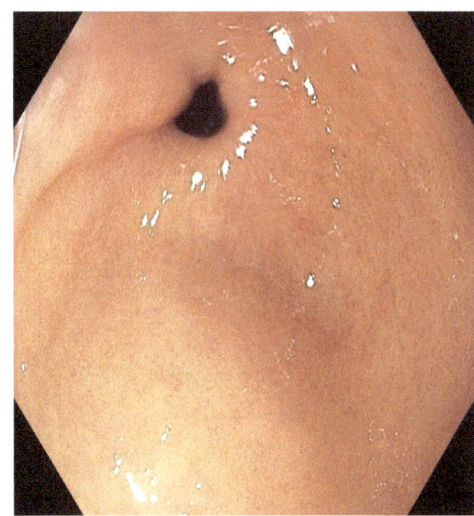

Figure 5.30

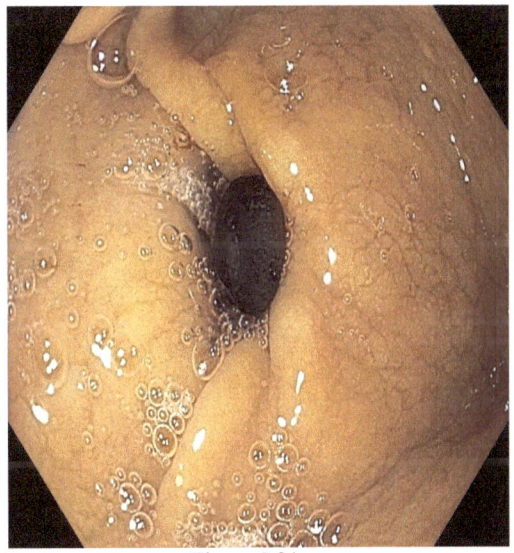

Figure 5.31

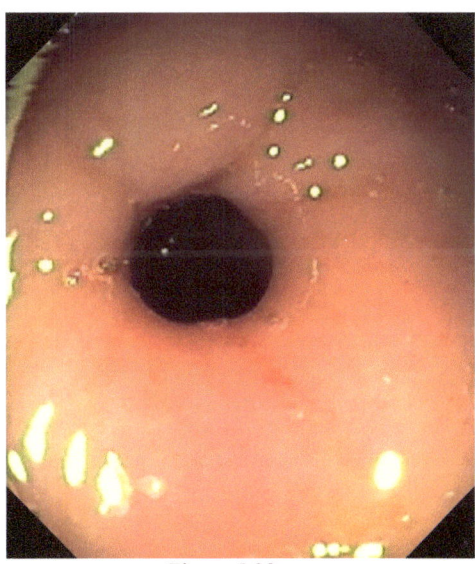

Figure 5.32

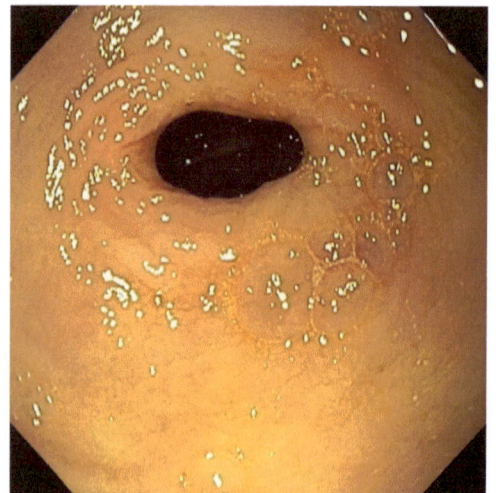
Figure 5.33

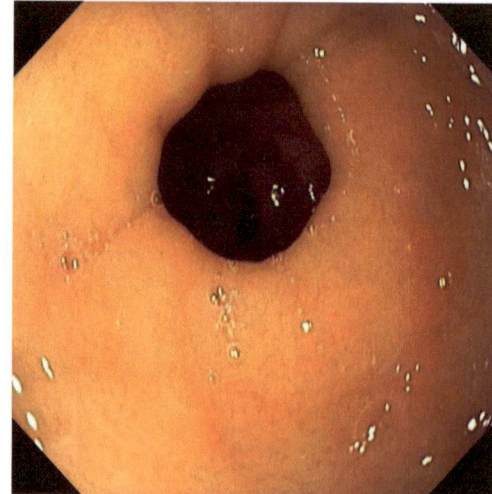
Figure 5.34

Gastric Cardia and Fundus

In other to have a complete view of these parts of the stomach, there is need to retroflex the scope at the level of the incisura. In the retroflexed position, the body and incisura are also examined fully. Whenever, the scope is in a retroflexed position, the shaft of the scope is always visible. Adjacent to the cardia and fundus are the diaphragm, spleen and heart, and the impressions of these organs and cardiac pulsation are visible in these parts of the stomach. Sometimes, a small pool of fluid can also be seen in the fundus.

Gastric Cardia

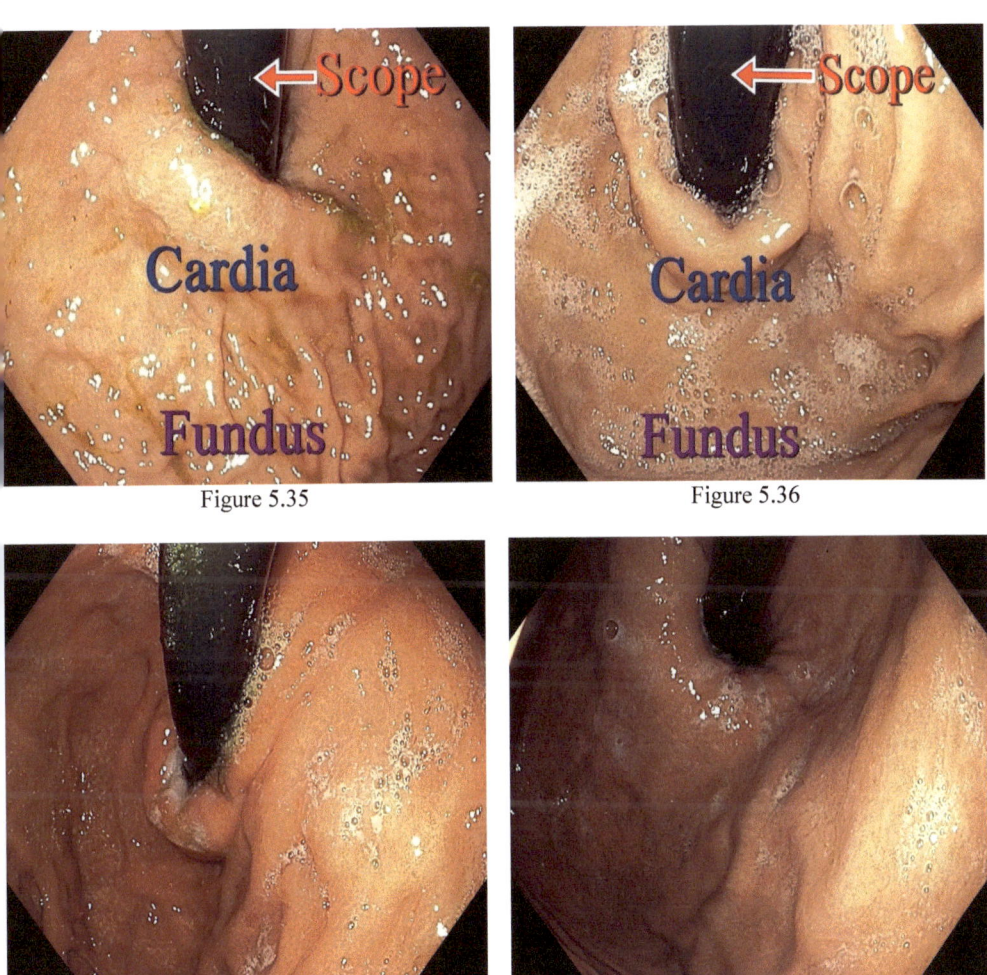

Figure 5.35

Figure 5.36

Figure 5.37

Figure 5.38

Gastric Fundus

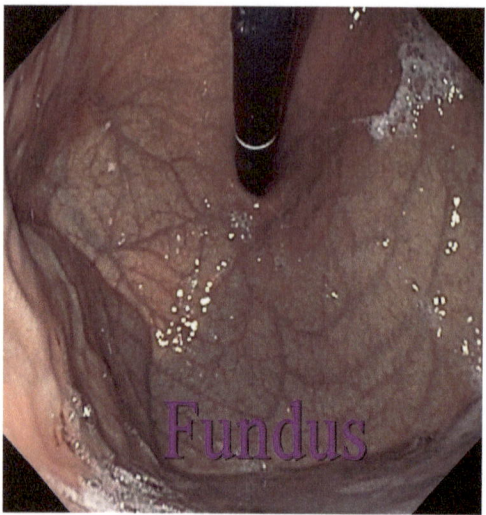

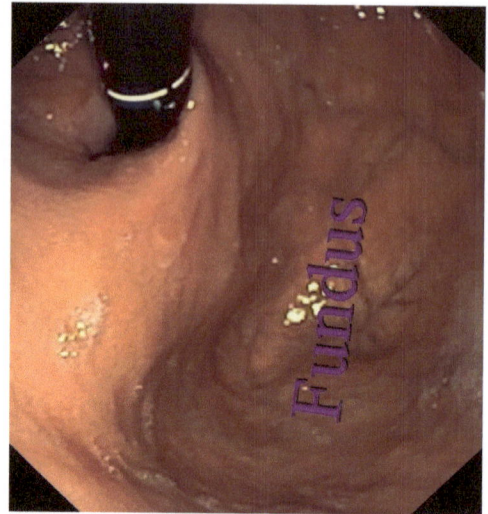

Figure 5.39
Splenic (blue) indentation & fluid in the fundus

Figure 5.40

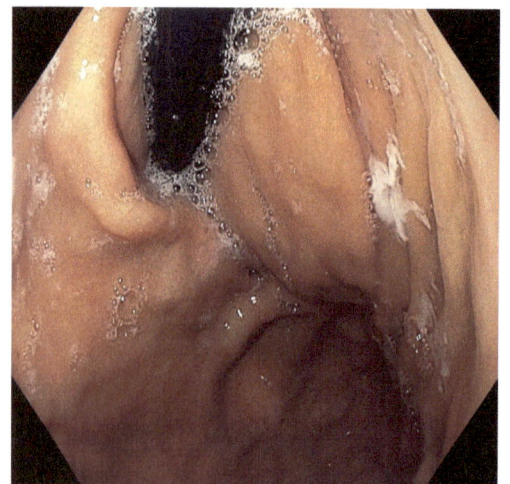

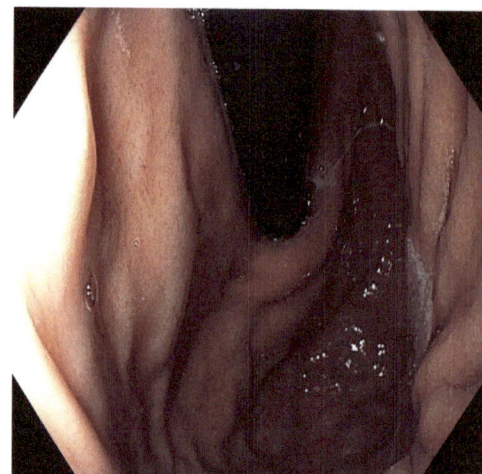

Figure 5.41

Figure 5.42

GASTRIC ABNORMALITIES

CHAPTER 6

Gastritis

It represents the reactions of the mucosa to the effects of noxious agents which could be bacteria (*H. pylori*); drugs (NSAIDs, steroids); bile; mechanical (foreign body, NG tube); vasculopathies; idiopathic. Gastritis could be acute or chronic. At endoscopy, features that suggest gastritis are:

- Mucosal erythema (Figures 6.1- 6.4)
- Mucosal oedema (Figures 6.5 & 6.6)
- Exudates
- Erosions (Figures 6.7- 6.10)
- Mucosal haemorrhagic lesions (Figures 6.11 - 6.14)

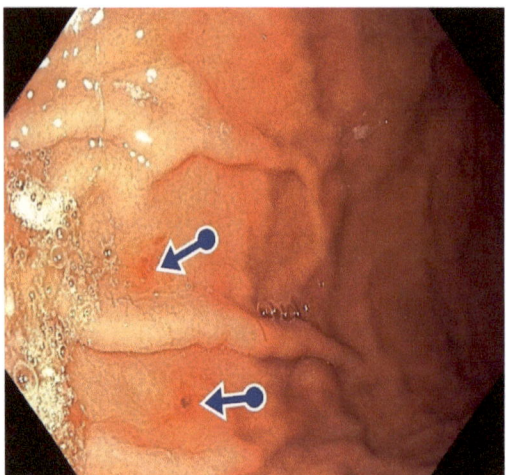

Figure 6.1:Mucosal erythema in the gastric body

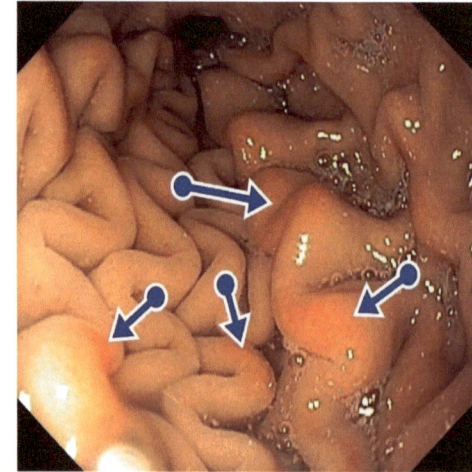

Figure 6.2: Mucosal erythema in the gastric body

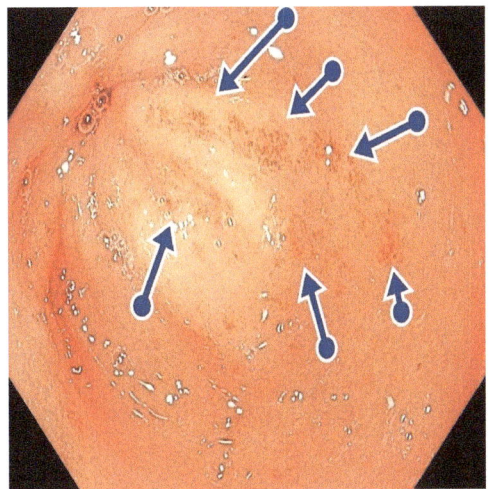
Figure 6.3: Mucosal erythema in the antrum

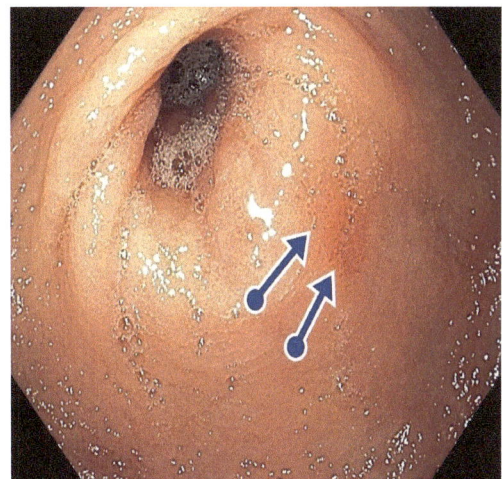
Figure 6.4: Mucosal erythema in the antrum

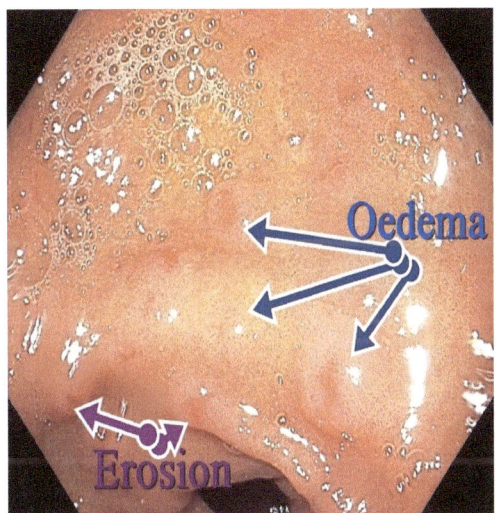
Figure 6.5: Mucosal oedema with erosions (antrum)

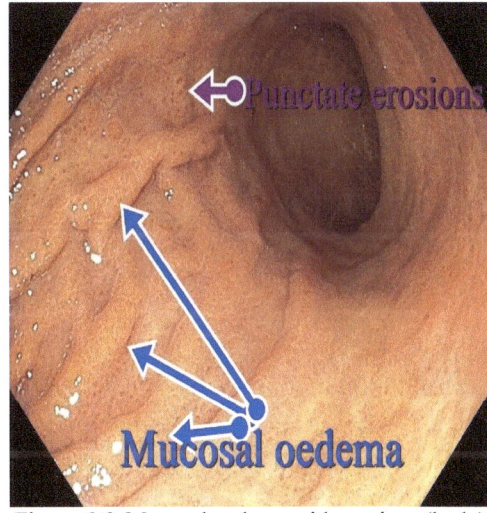
Figure 6.6: Mucosal oedema with erosions (body)

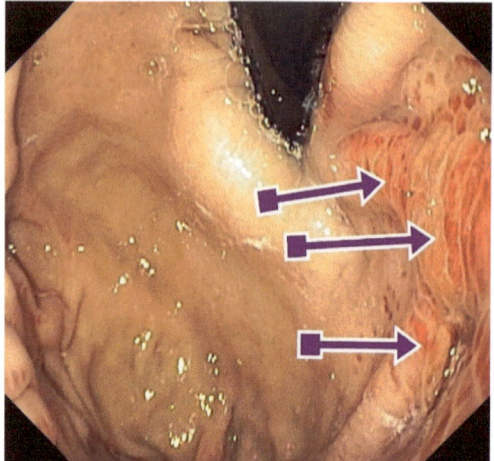
Figure 6.7: Erosions in the cardia

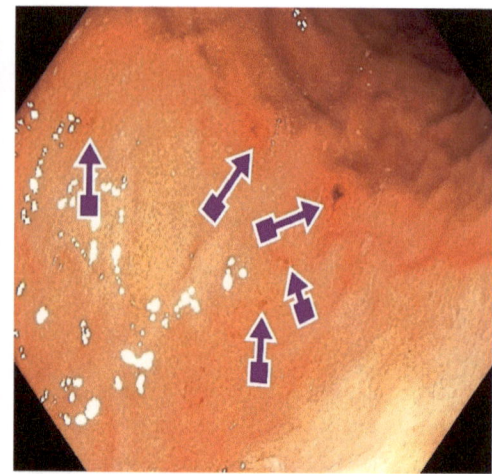
Figure 6.8: Erosions in the body

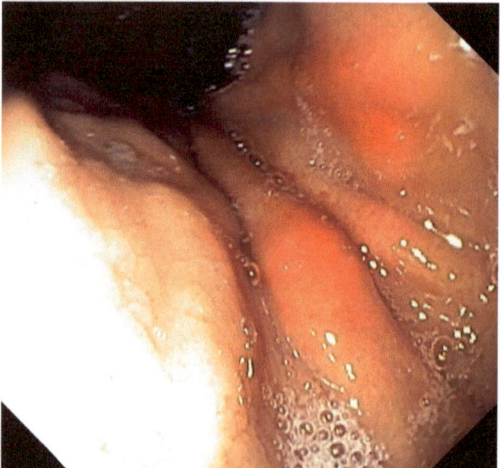
Figure 6.9: Erosions and mucosal oedema (body)

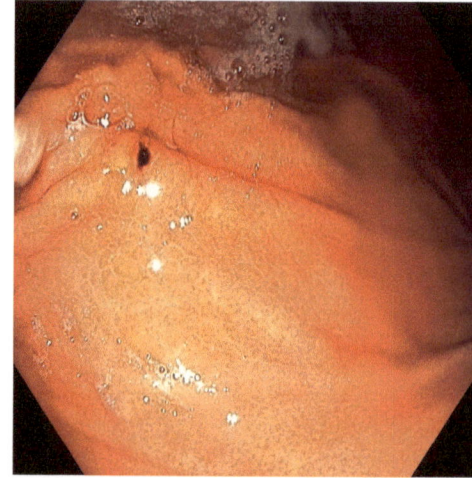
Figure 6.10: Erosion and mucosal oedema (body)

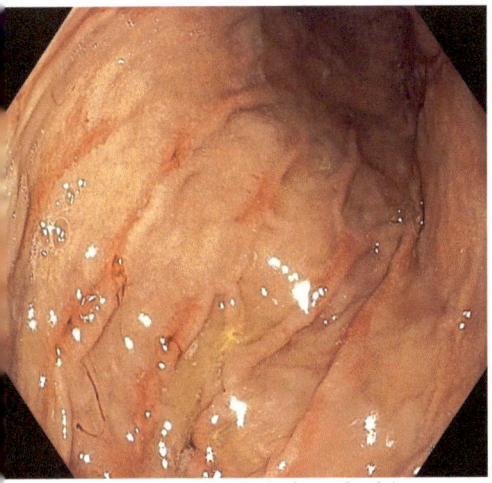
Figure 6.11: Haemorrhagic lesions (body)

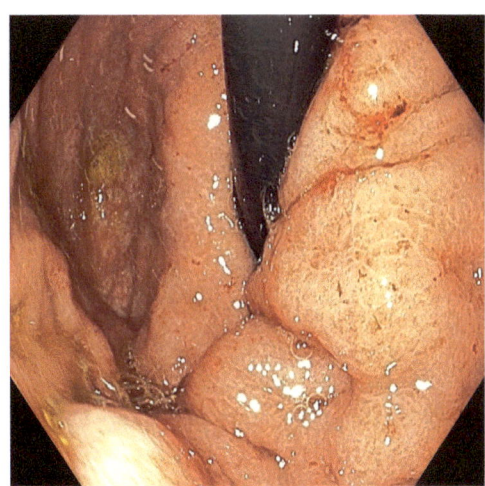
Figure 6.12: Haemorrhagic lesions (cardia)

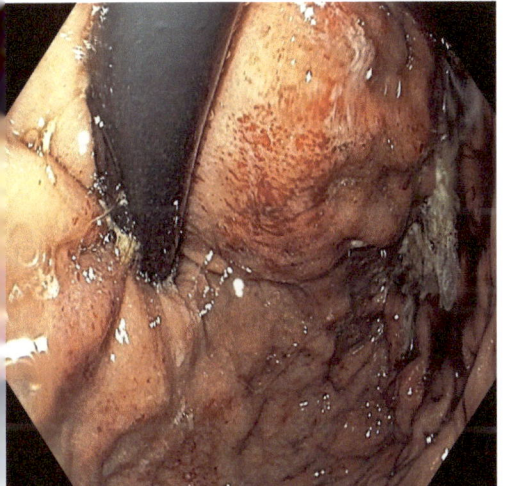
Figure 6.13: Haemorrhagic lesions (cardia, fundus)

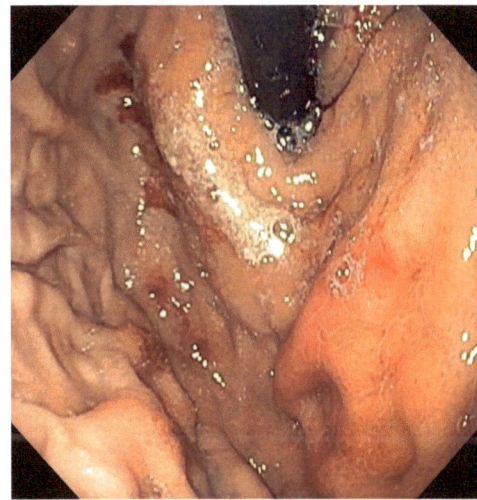
Figure 6.14: Haemorrhagic lesions (cardia, fundus)

Gastric Ulcer

It is a mucosal defect that extends into the submucosal layer. The two most important precipitating factors are non-steroidal anti-inflammatory drugs (NSAIDs) and *Helicobacter pylori* (*H. pylori*). The latter is responsible for about 70% of cases of gastric ulcer.

Ulcers can be found in any part of the stomach, but in about 80% of cases, they are found in the antrum or at the incisura along the lesser curve.

The description of an ulcer at endoscopy should include the following:

- Location
- Number
- Size: You can estimate this using the cups of an open biopsy forceps, the diameter of the cups of most biopsy forceps is about 5 mm
- Shape: linear, oval, irregular, round
- Edge: raised, flat
- Base: This should be described using the Forrest grades:
  - Grade Ia: Spurting haemorrhage at the base
  - Grade Ib: Oozing haemorrhage at the base
  - Grade IIa: Non-bleeding visible vessel at the base
  - Grade IIb: Adherent clot at the base
  - Grade IIc: Pigmented spot at the base
  - Grade III: Clean base ulcer

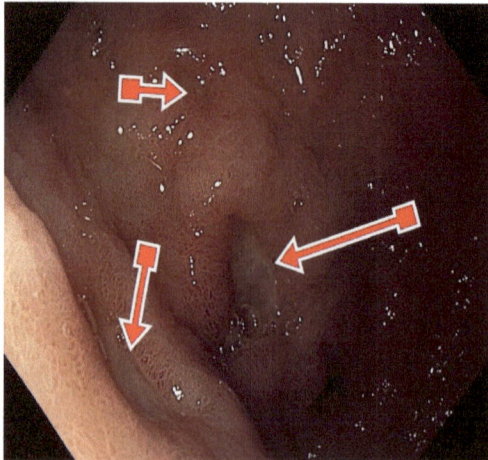

Figure 6.15
Multiple clean base antral ulcers (Forrest III)

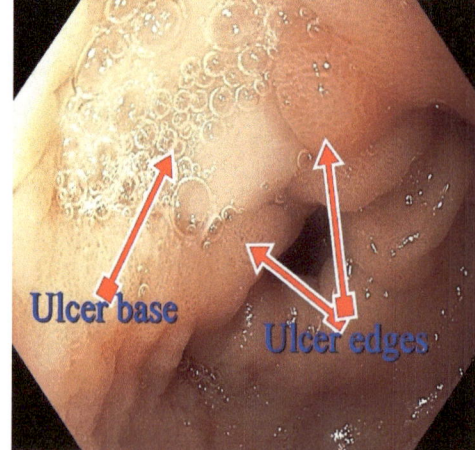

Figure 6.16
Clean base prepyloric ulcer (Forrest III)

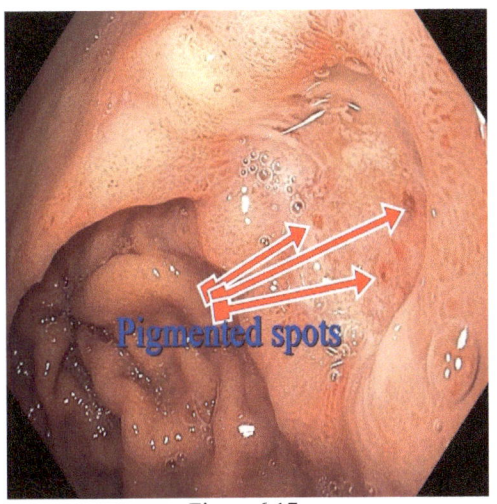

Figure 6.17
Antral ulcer with pigmented spots (Forrest IIc)

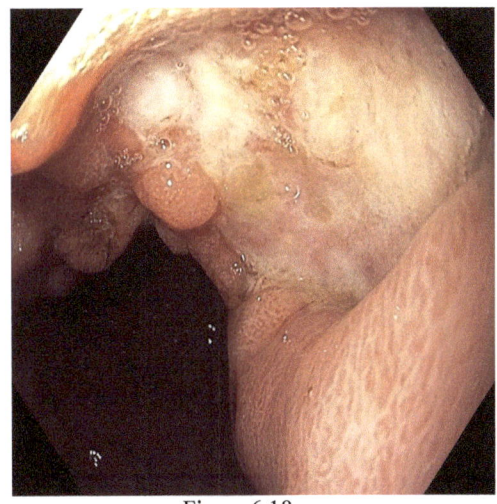

Figure 6.18
Antral ulcer on the greater curve with raised edges

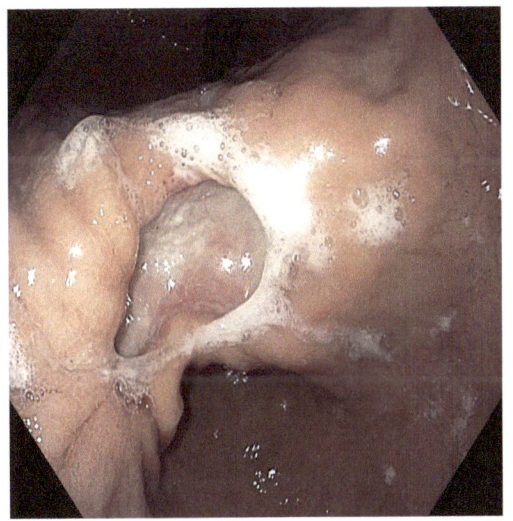

Figure 6.19
Ulcer at the incisura (note the raised edges)

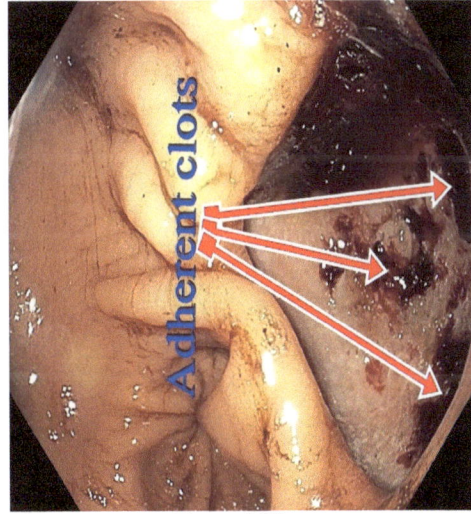

Figure 6.20
Antral ulcer with adherent clots (Forrest IIb)

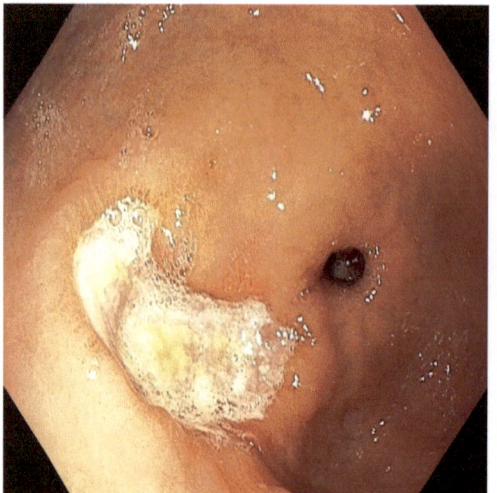
Figure 6.21: Prepyloric clean base ulcer

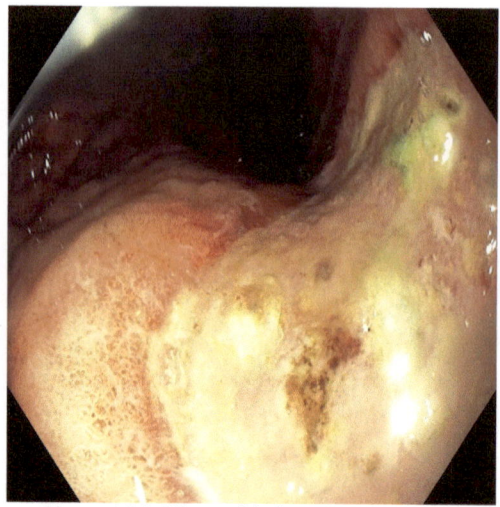
Figure 6.22: Ulcer with flat edges in the body

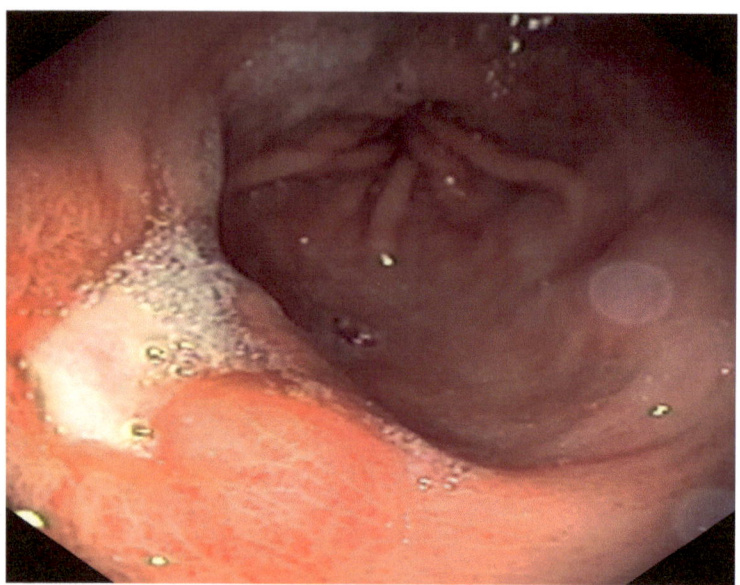
Figure 6.23
Clean base ulcer at the incisura with flat edges and surrounding inflammation

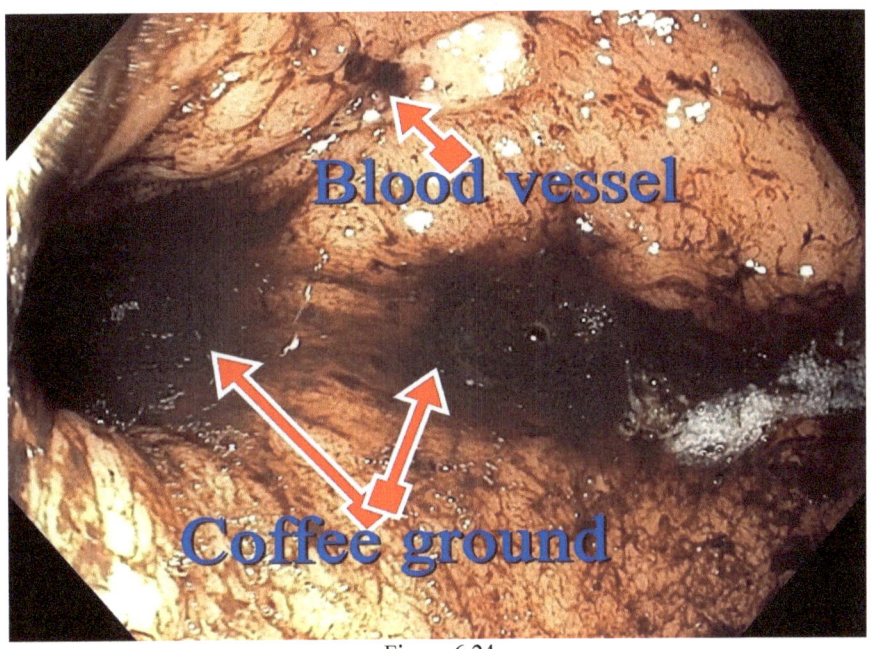

Figure 6.24
Ulcer in the body (Posterior wall) with non-bleeding visible vessel at the base (Forrest IIa)
Note: Coffee ground material in the lumen

Gastric Varices

About 20% of patients with portal hypertension have gastric varices, and about 5-10% of them have isolated gastric varices (no accompanying oesophageal varices). Endoscopic recognition of gastric varices is more difficult compared to oesophageal varices. They sometimes can be mistaken for a mucosal fold when small or for a tumour, and biopsy of this can be disastrous. However at endoscopy gastric varices resemble clusters of grape with bluish tinge. Gastric varices are classified as follows:

- ➢ Gastroesophageal varices type 1 (GOV 1) when oesophageal varices extend to the lesser curve
- ➢ Gastroesophageal varices type 2 (GOV 2) when oesophageal varices extend to the greater curve
- ➢ Isolated gastric varices type 1 (IGV 1) are located in the fundus
- ➢ Isolated gastric varices type 2 (IGV 2) are located in other parts of the stomach or first part of the duodenum.

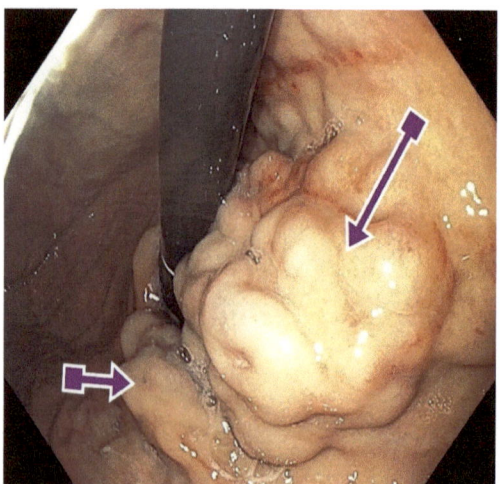

Figure 6.25: GOV 1

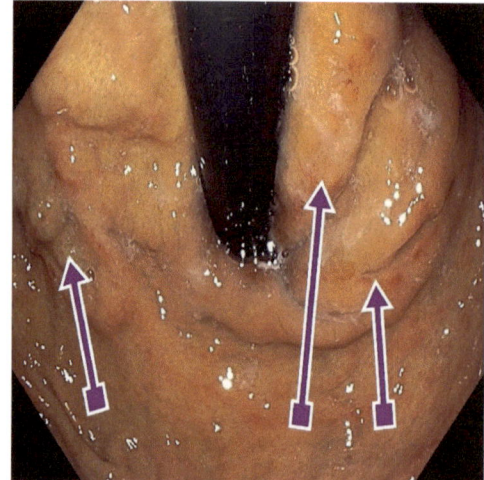

Figure 6.26: GOV 1

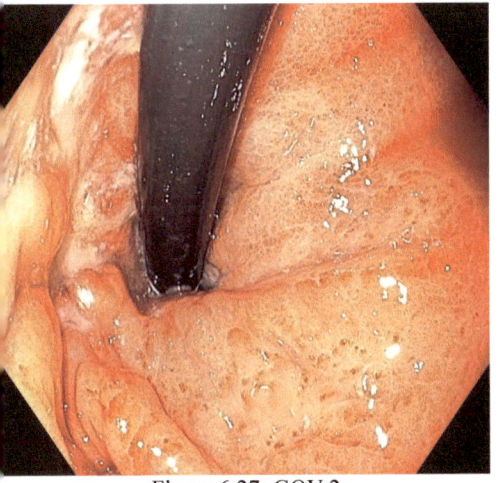
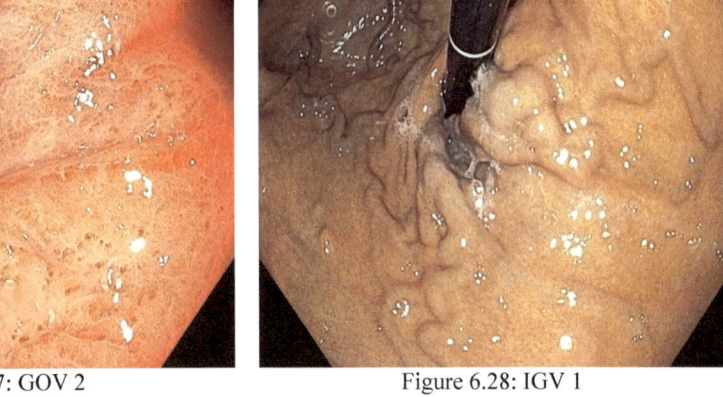

Figure 6.27: GOV 2   Figure 6.28: IGV 1

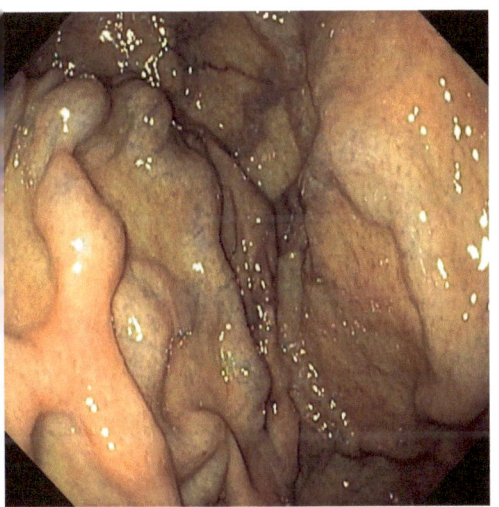
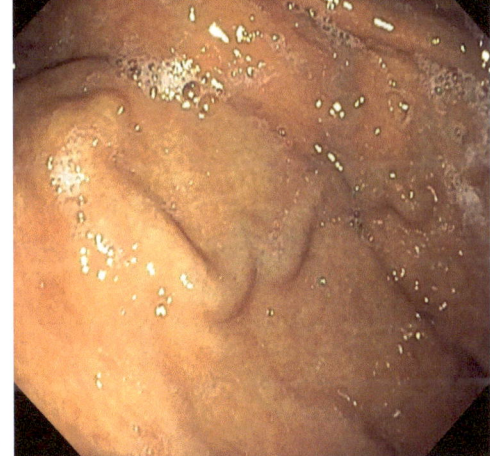

Figure 6.29: IGV 1   Figure 6.30: IGV 1

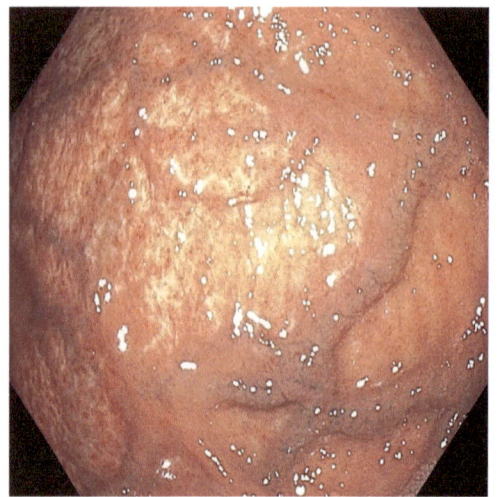
Figure 6.31: IGV 1

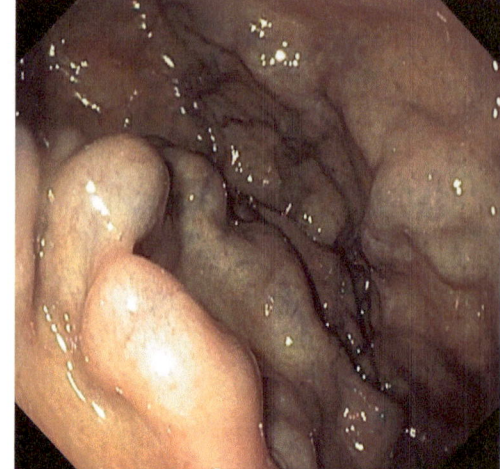
Figure 6.32: IGV 1

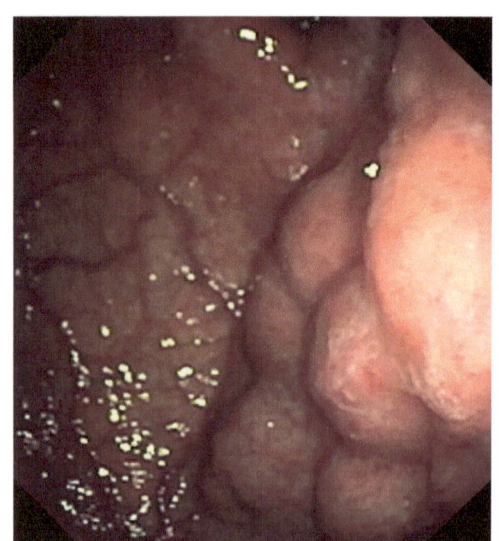
Figure 6.33: IGV 1

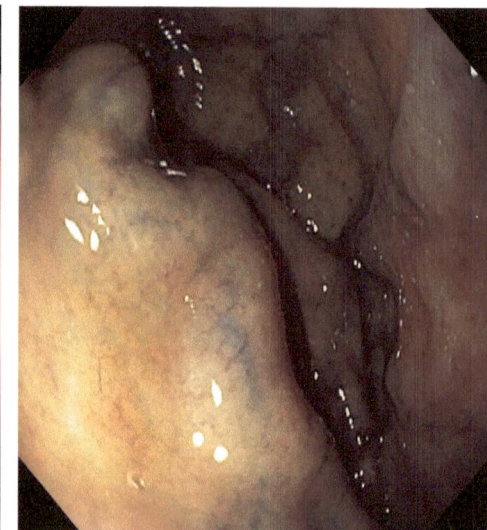
Figure 6.34: IGV 1

Portal Hypertensive Gastropathy (PHG)

Portal hypertensive gastropathy is seen in patients with portal hypertension of any cause. The mucosa of the stomach has mosaic pattern with or without accompanying widespread erosions. On endoscopy, it appears as reticular network which is separated by raised red or pink areas, resembling 'snake skin'

Portal hypertensive gastropathy is most pronounced in the fundus and body of the stomach, but can be seen in the antrum. These changes can also occur in the small and large intestines.

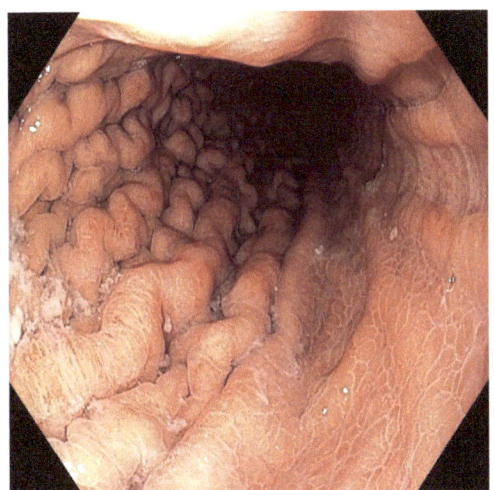

Figure 6.35: Snake-skin appearance of the mucosa

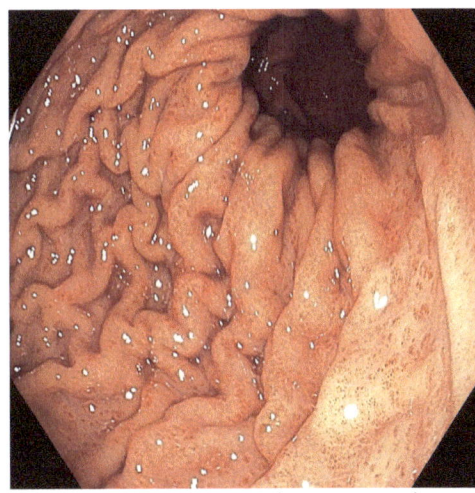

Figure 6.36: Widespread punctate erosions

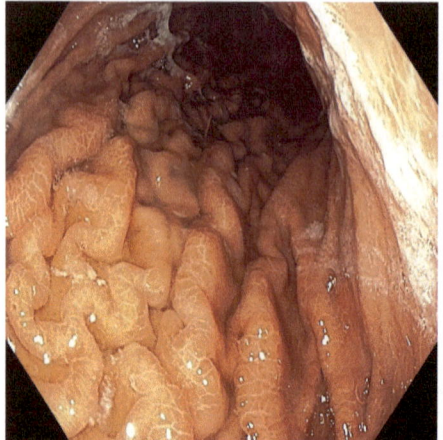
Figure 6.37: Snake-skin appearance of the mucosa

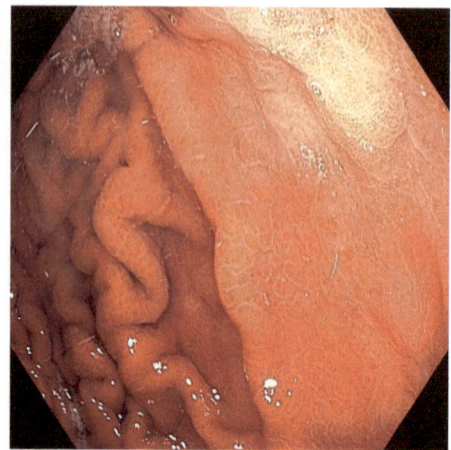
Figure 6.38: Snake-skin appearance of the mucosa

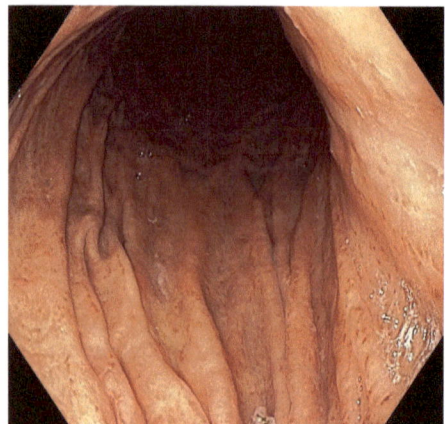
Figure 6.39: Widespread punctate erosions

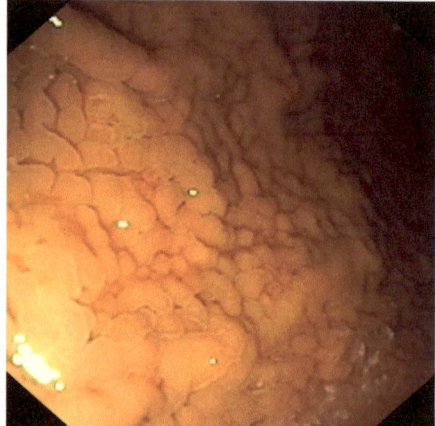
Figure 6.40: Snake-skin appearance of the mucosa

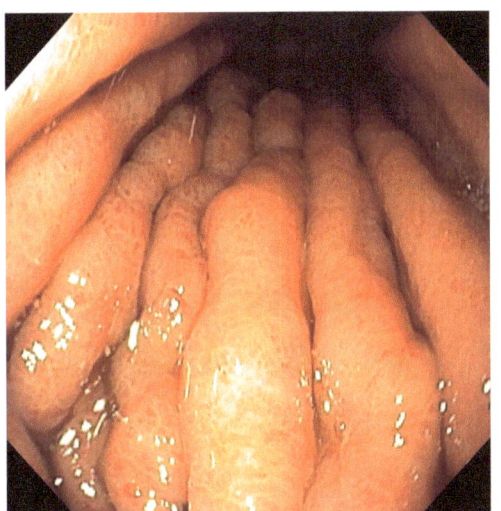
Figure 6.41
Mucosa oedema with punctate erosions (Body)

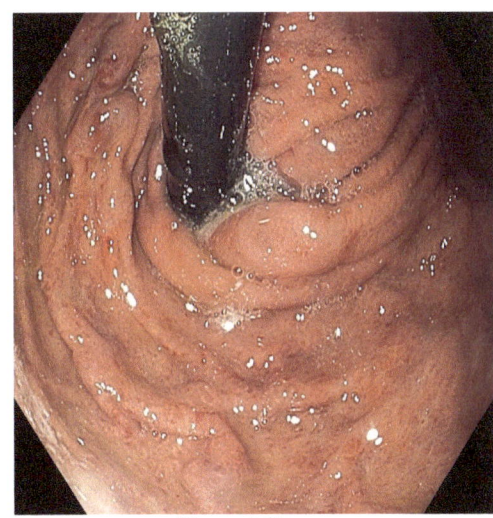
Figure 6.42
Oedema with punctate erosions (Cardia & Fundus)

Gastric Cancer

Gastric cancer is the second leading cause of cancer death in the world after lung cancer. About 90% of gastric cancers are adenocarcinoma, the rest are non-Hodgkin's lymphoma (NHL) and leiomyosarcoma. Less than 20% of gastric cancers are diagnosed at an early stage in low risk areas, whereas, the incidence of early gastric cancer is about 40-50% in high risk areas like Japan. Detection of early gastric cancer requires high index of suspicion and low threshold for endoscopy.

Thorough inspection of the entire gastric mucosa should be carried out by fully distending the stomach during gastroscopy, and view the cardia and fundus by retroflexion. Early gastric cancer can present as areas of:

- pallor or erythema
- nodularity
- depression
- ulceration
- protrusion

Such areas should be biopsied. However, most patients present with advanced disease. About 50% of the lesions are located in the antrum, and 25% in the body.
At endoscopy, advanced gastric cancer can be:

- ulcerated (Figures 6.43 - 6.45)
- polypoid (Figures 6.46 - 6.48)
- fungating (Figures 6.49 - 6.52)
- flat
- diffusely infiltrating the wall of the stomach (linitis plastic).

Fungating or ulcerated lesions are the most common (60-70%). Ulcerated gastric cancer may resemble benign ulcer, but the distinguishing features are:
- larger size
- shaggy or irregular base
- heaped up edges

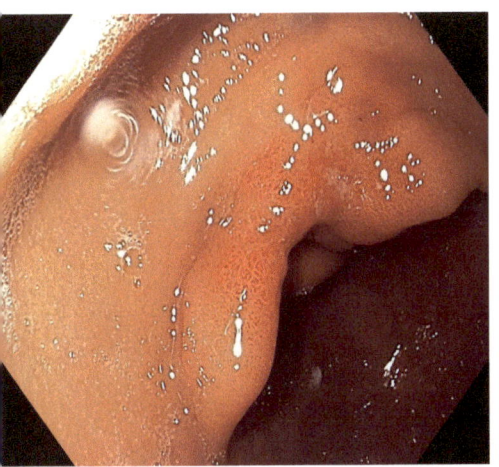

Figure 6.43

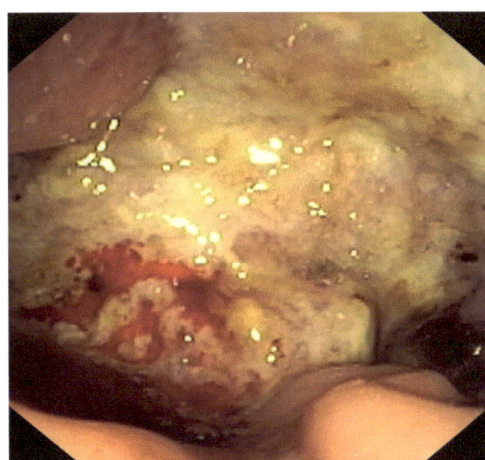

Figure 6.44

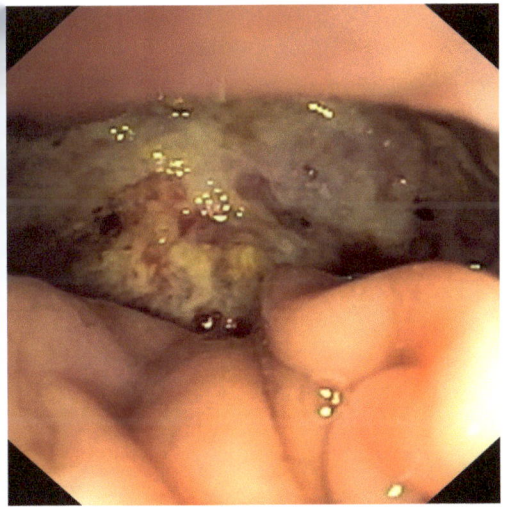

Figure 6.45

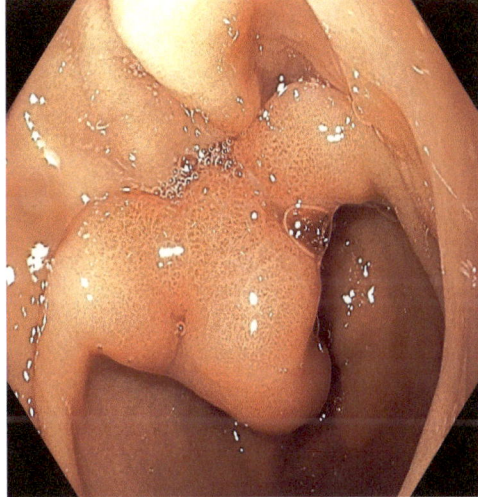

Figure 6.46

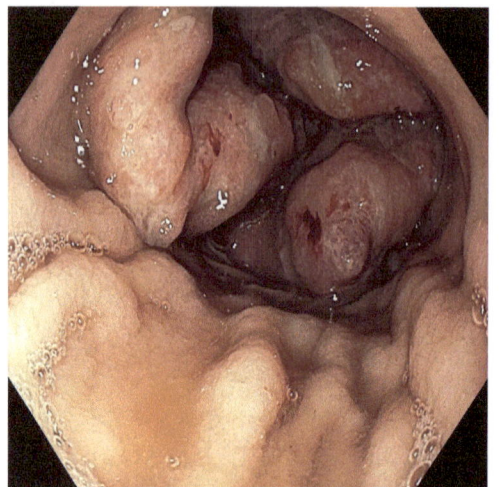

Figure 6.47

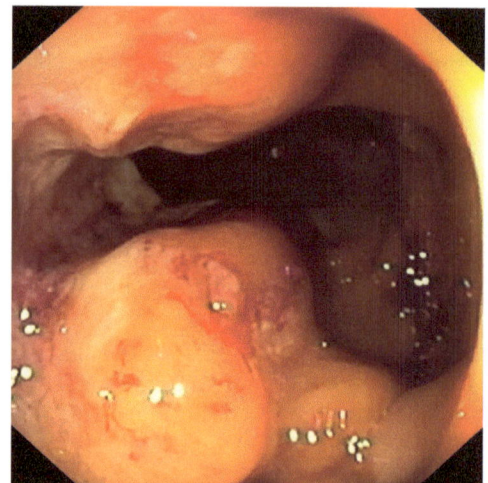

Figure 6.48

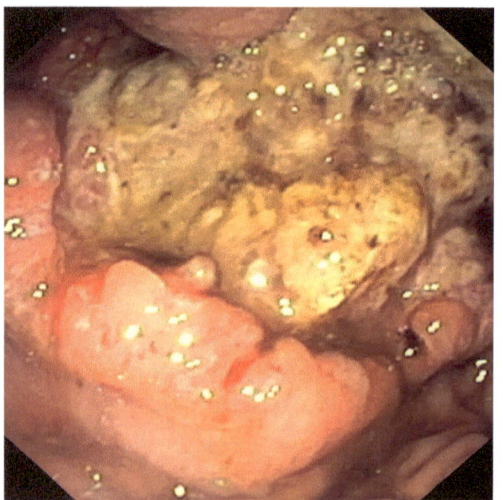

Figure 6.49

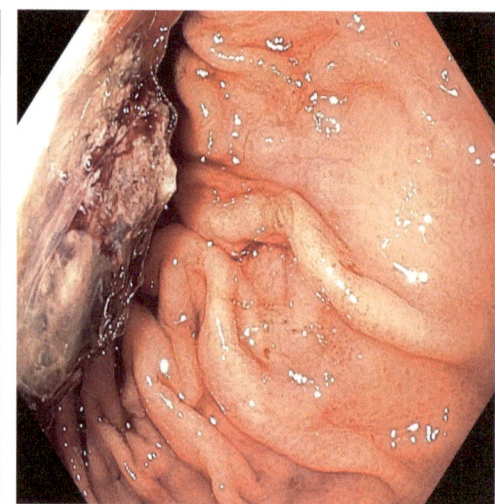

Figure 6.50

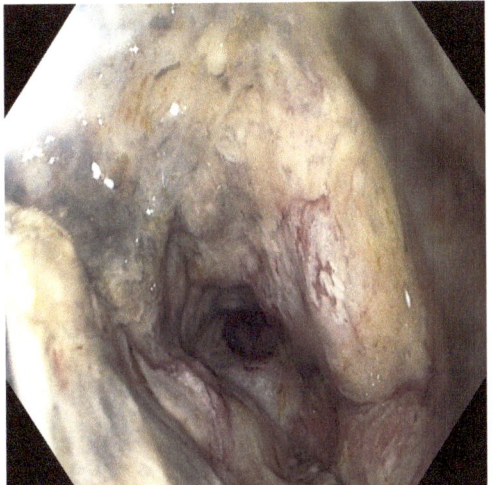

Figure 6.51

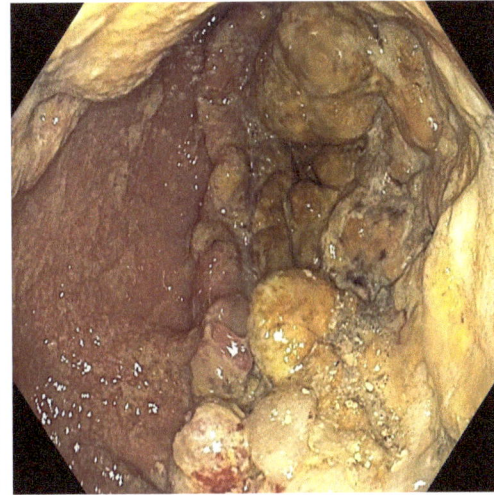

Figure 6.52

Gastrointestinal Stromal Tumours (GISTs)

Gastrointestinal stromal tumours originate in the mesenchymal stroma. They stain positive for CD117, which is a specific membrane protein called KIT (a tyrosine kinase receptor), which mediates cell proliferation and apoptotic cell death. Mutations in the associated proto-oncogene (c-KIT) lead to changes in the membrane kinase and eventual abnormal cell growth. Most GISTs are found in the stomach, but some have been described in the duodenum.

At endoscopy, GISTs have the following features:

- ✓ usually solitary
- ✓ mostly <3cm in size, but size of 10 cm has been described
- ✓ submucosal in nature and firm
- ✓ dome-shaped
- ✓ may have irregular or lobulated contour
- ✓ may be ulcerated or have central umbilication

GISTs grow slowly, but there is a risk of being malignant. Based on this potential, they are classified into:

- ➤ benign
- ➤ indeterminate/uncertain
- ➤ malignant

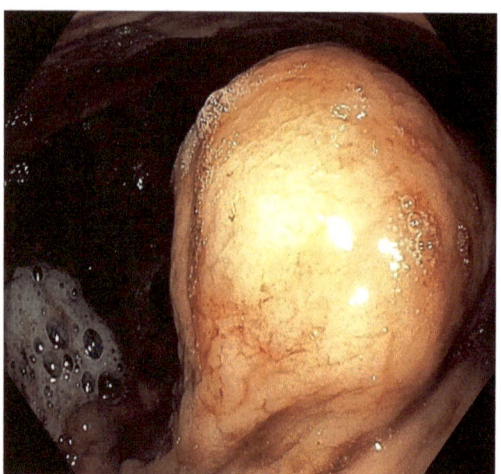

Figure 6.53

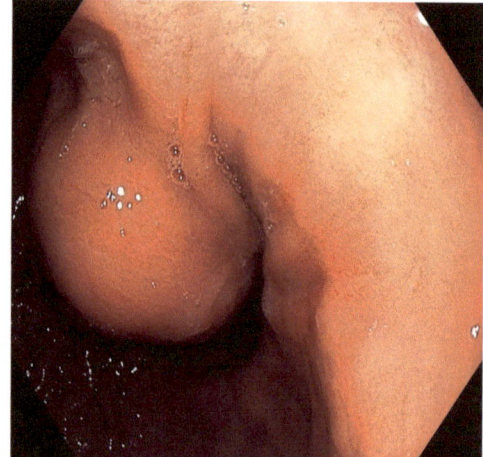

Figure 6.54

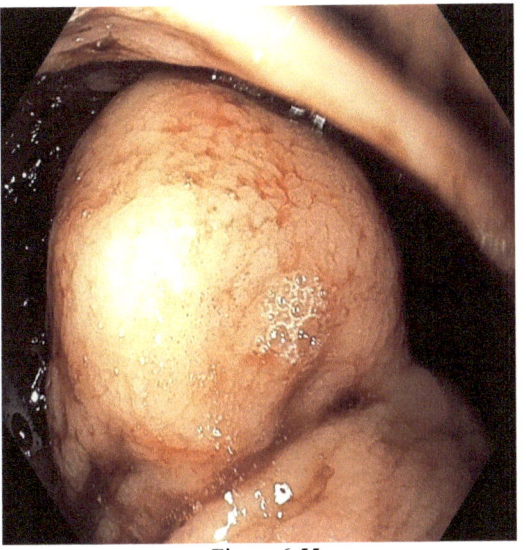

Figure 6.55

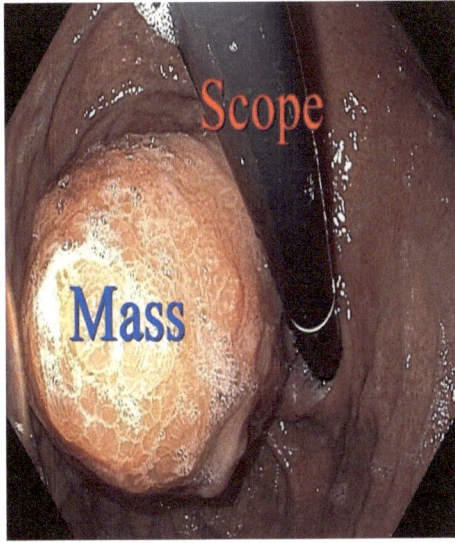

Figure 6.56

Other Gastric Abnormalities

Figure 6.57: Pyloric stenosis
Figure 6.58: Gastric Polyps
Figure 6.59: Gastric Angiodysplasia
Figure 6.60: Coffee-ground material in the stomach in a patient with recent Upper Gastrointestinal Bleeding

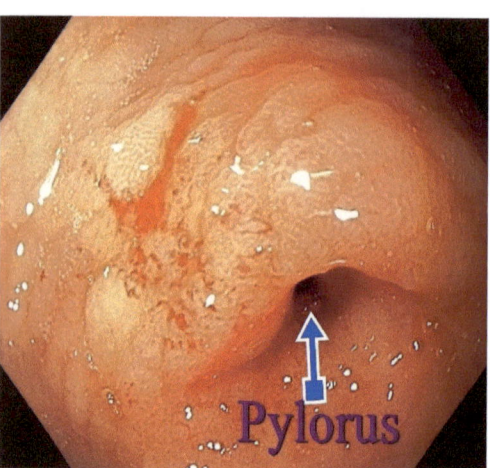

Figure 6.57

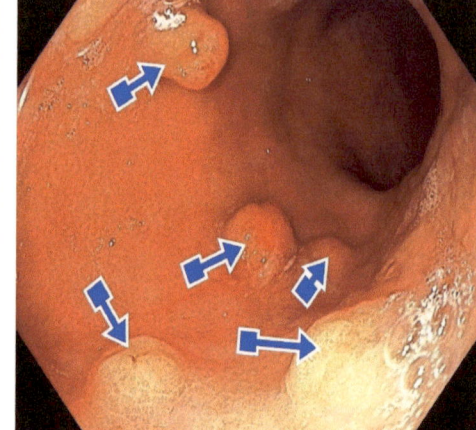

Figure 6.58

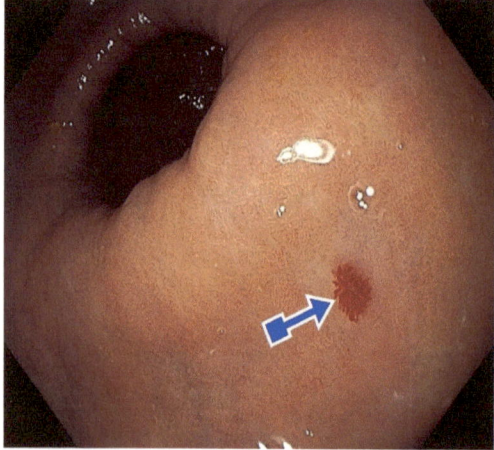

Figure 6.59

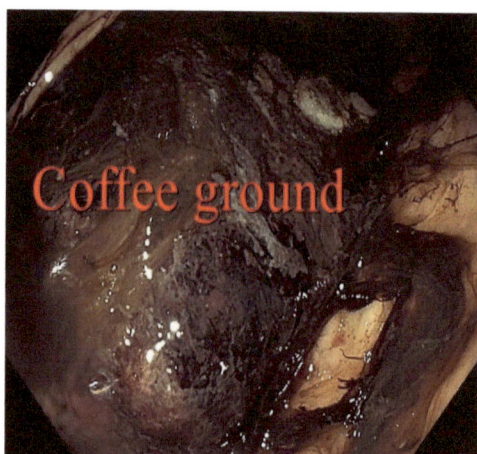

Figure 6.60

Figure 6.61: Blood clots in the stomach in a patient with Upper Gastrointestinal Bleeding
Figure 6.62: Faeces in the stomach in a patient with gastrocolic fistula

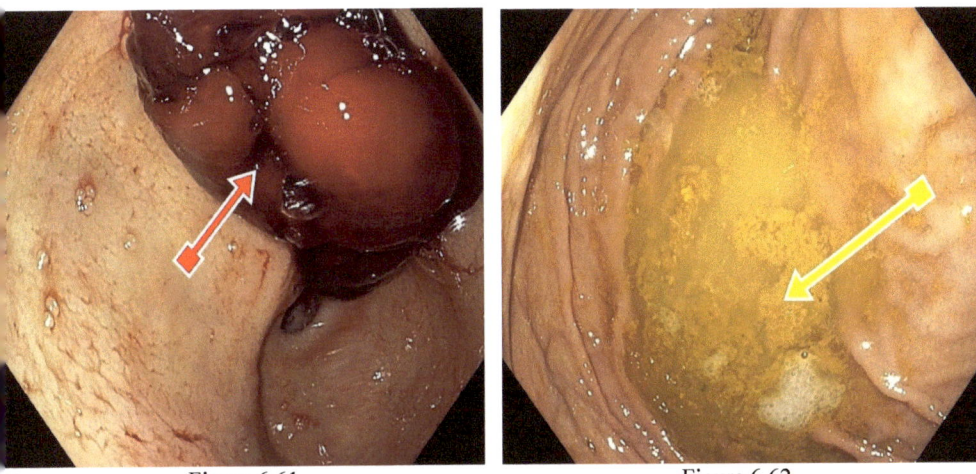

Figure 6.61　　　　　　　　　　　　　　Figure 6.62

Figures 6.63 & 6.64 are gastric devices employed for feeding of patients
Figure 6.63: Nasogastric Tube in the stomach
Figure 6.64: Balloon and distal end of a Percutaneous Gastrostomy Tube

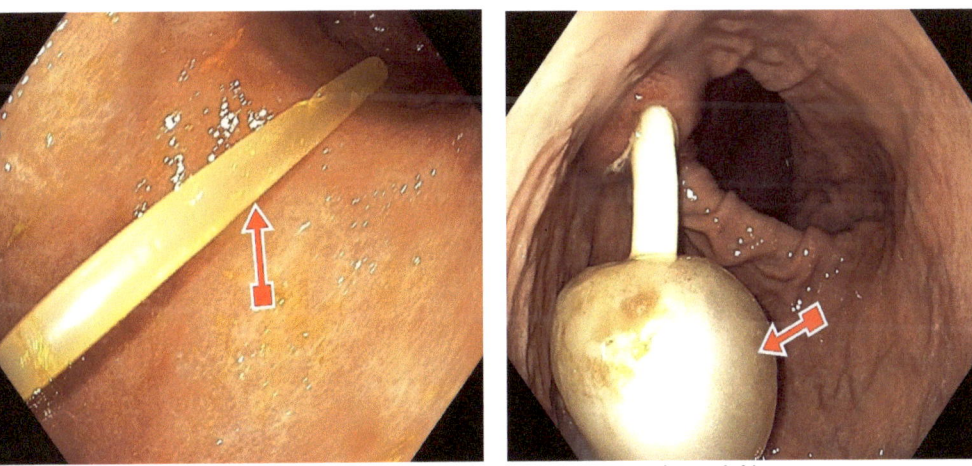

Figure 6.63　　　　　　　　　　　　　　Figure 6.64

DUODENUM

CHAPTER 7

Normal Duodenum

The duodenum is the first segment of the small intestine. It consists of 4 parts:

- Superior duodenum (Duodenal bulb, Duodenal cap or D1)
- Descending duodenum (D2)
- Horizontal (Inferior) duodenum (D3)
- Ascending duodenum (D4)

During upper gastrointestinal endoscopy, the endoscope usually may not go beyond the D3.

Duodenal Bulb

It is the part seen immediately after the pylorus. Sometimes, a small pool of fluid may be seen within it. Endoscopically, it looks bulbous, but may be oblong or rounded. The surface is smooth, it lacks mucosal folds. It is yellowish-gray in colour and the villi may be visible on closer view.

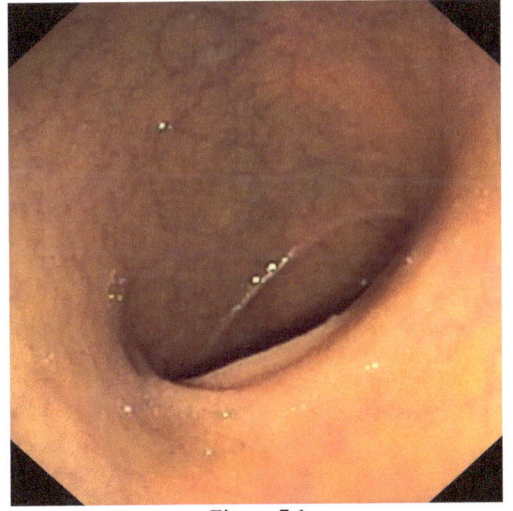

Figure 7.1   Figure 7.2

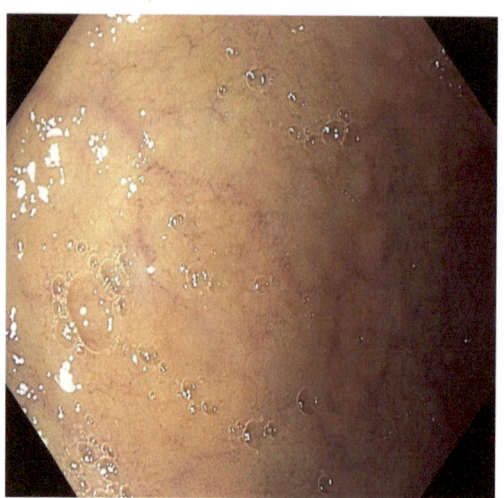

Figure 7.3

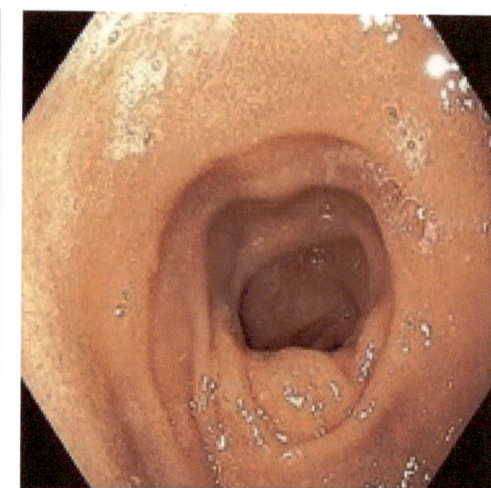

Figure 7.4

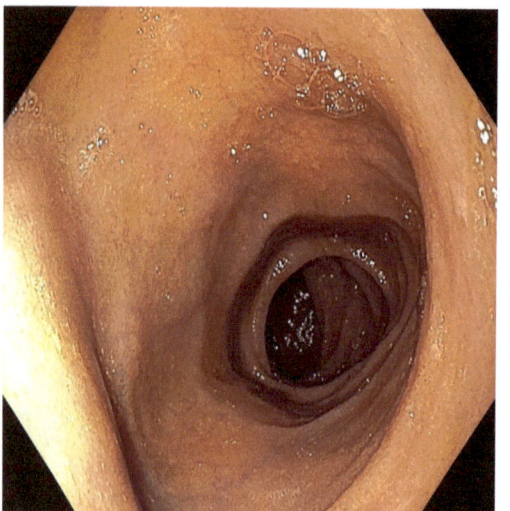

Figure 7.5

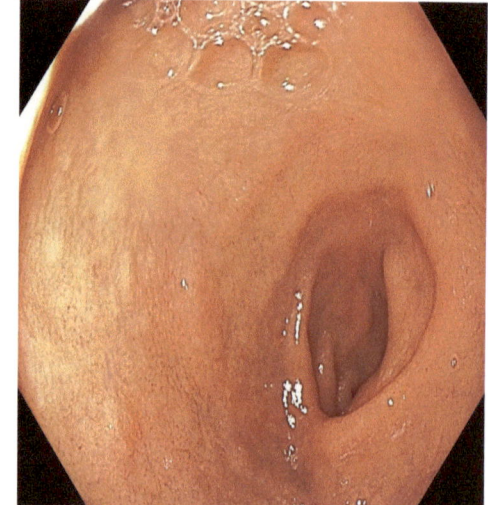

Figure 7.6

Descending Duodenum

This is the second part of the duodenum after the bulb. It has an appearance of a curved tunnel. It has circular folds called valvulae conniventes and finely granular mucosa. Located in this part of the duodenum are the major and minor papillae.

The major papilla (papilla of Vater) is usually more visible than the minor papilla. The papilla of Vater is usually seen at 9 or 10 O'clock of the endoscopic view. However, it is difficult to adequately evaluate the papillae with a forward-viewing endoscope.

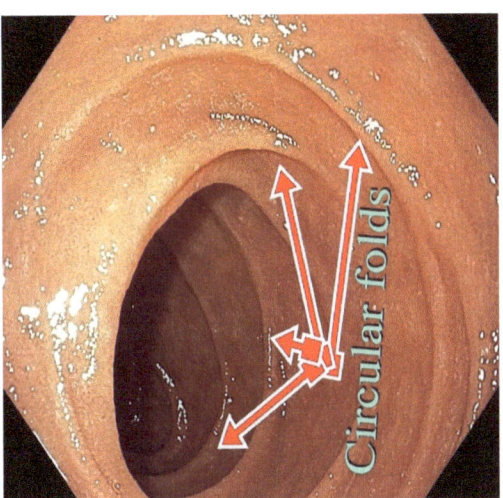

Figure 7.7

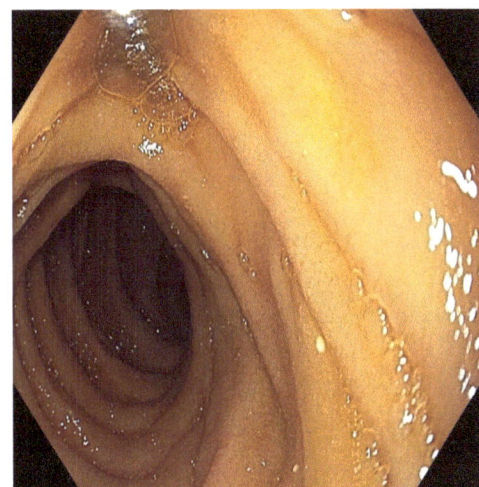

Figure 7.8

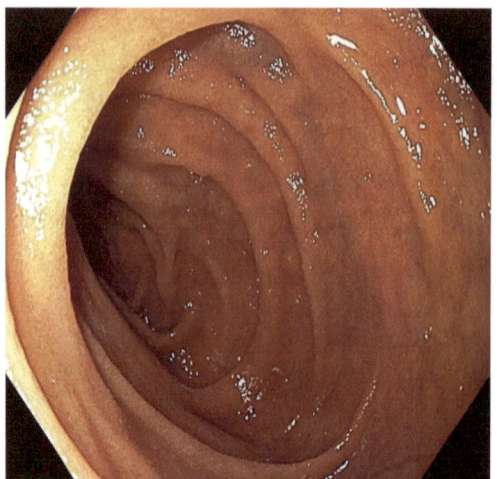
Figure 7.9

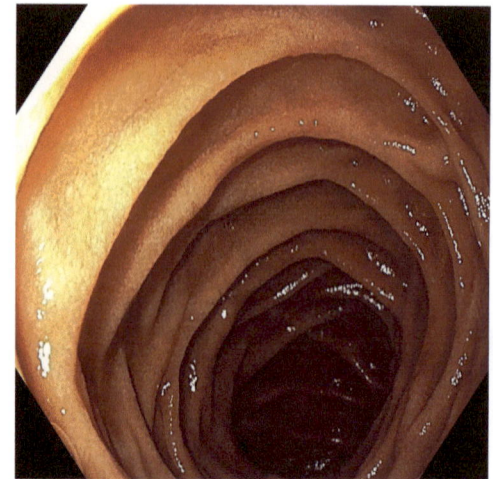
Figure 7.10

Descending Duodenum with Papilla of Vater (Figures 7.11 - 7.16)

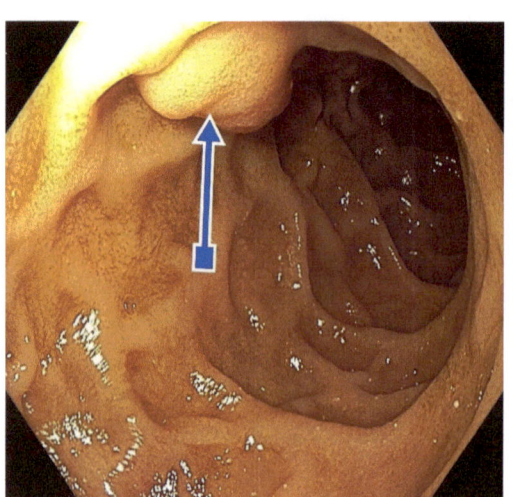
Figure 7.11

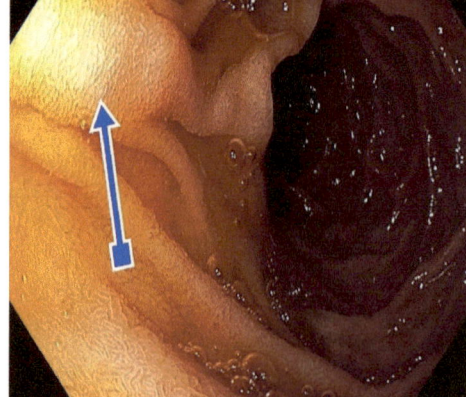
Figure 7.12

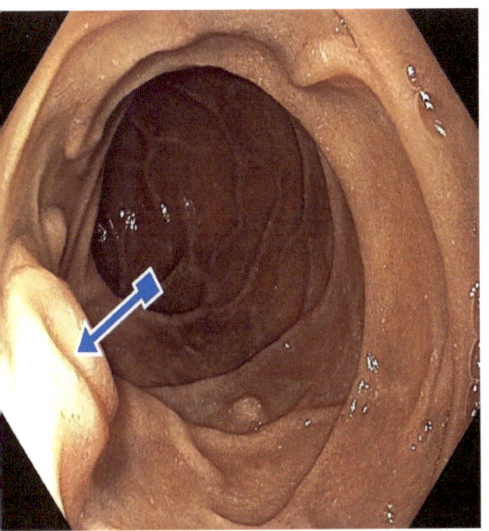

Figure 7.13

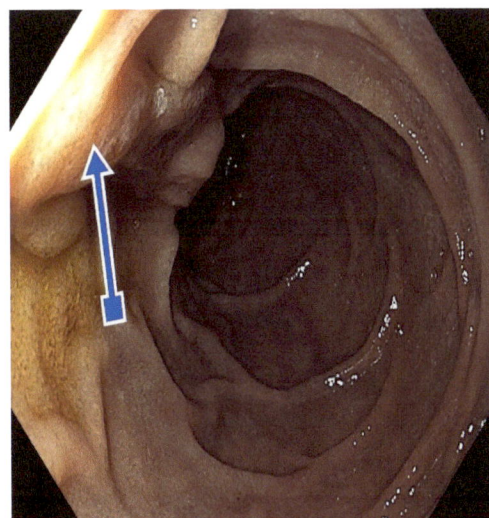

Figure 7.14

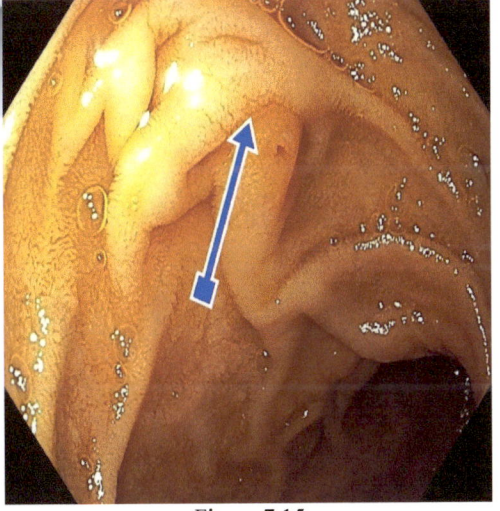

Figure 7.15

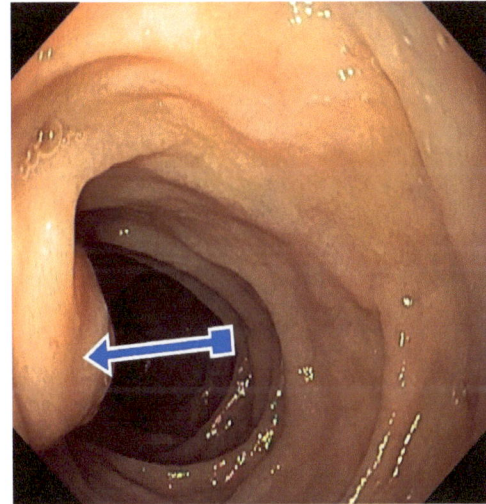

Figure 7.16

Horizontal (Inferior) Duodenum

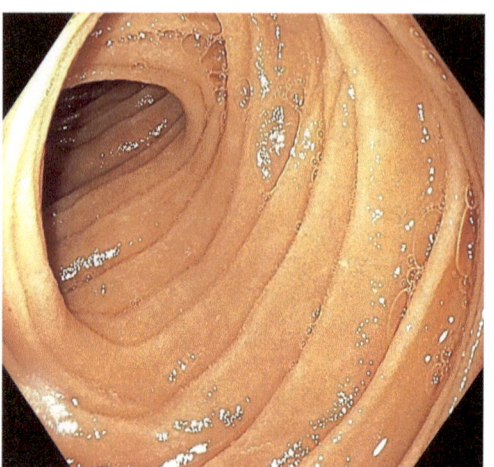

Figure 7.17

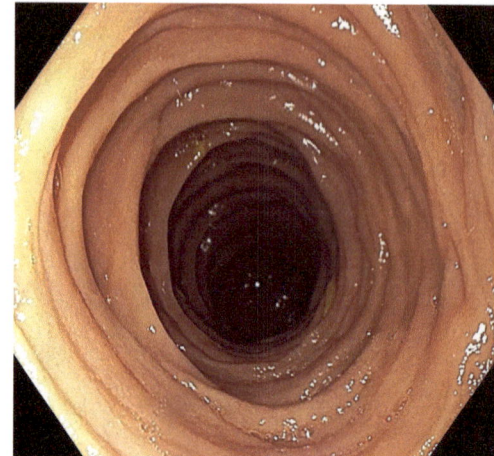

Figure 7.18

DUODENAL ABNORMALITIES

CHAPTER 8

Duodenitis

This is an inflammation of the mucosa of the duodenum. At endoscopy, it is characterized by:

- ✓ Mucosal oedema
- ✓ Mucosal erythema
- ✓ Raised or flat erosions

These lesions could be patchy, spotty or diffuse in distribution.

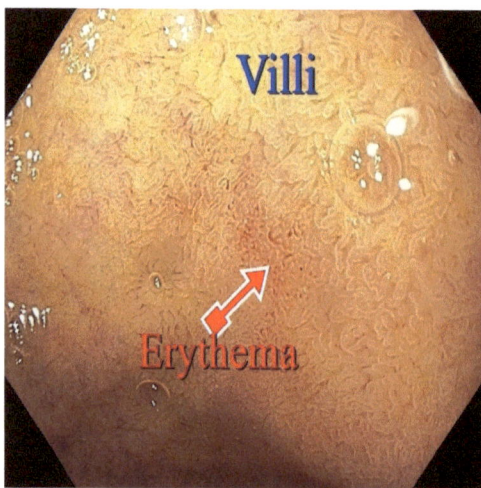

Figure 8.1: Spotty erythema

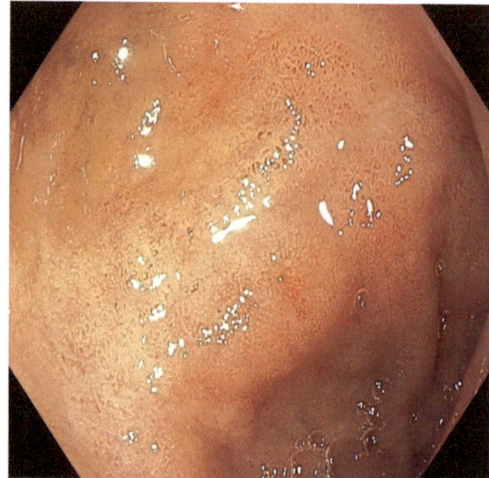

Figure 8.2: Patchy erythema and oedema

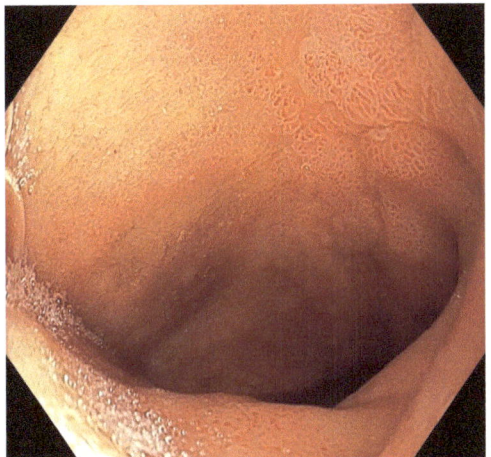
Figure 8.3: Patchy erythema and oedema

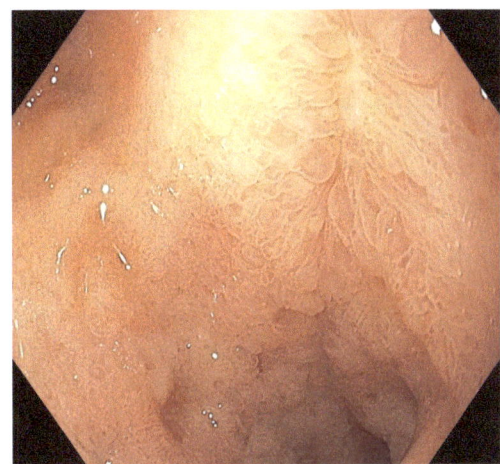
Figure 8.4: Diffuse mucosal oedema

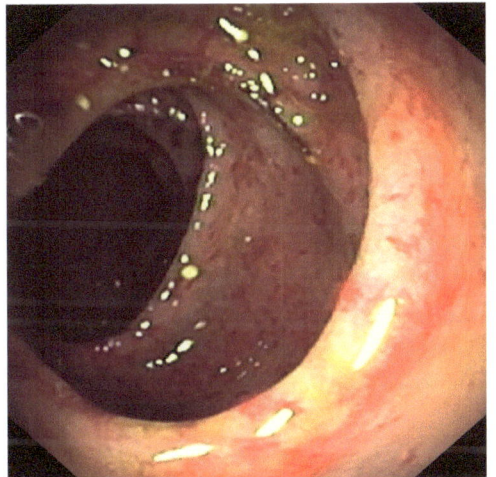
Figure 8.5: Diffuse mucosal erythema

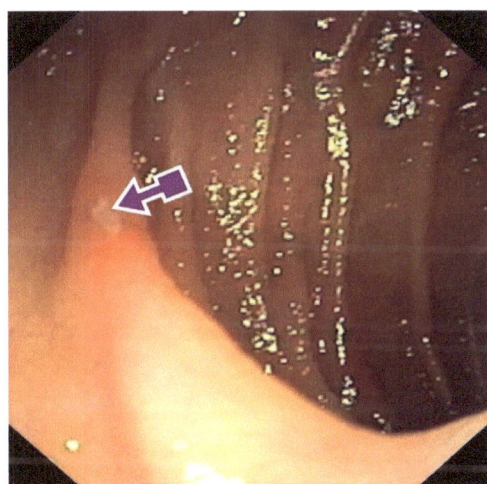
Figure 8.6: Erosion in the D2

Duodenal Ulcer

It is a mucosal defect that extends into the submucosa. About 90% of duodenal ulcers are located in the duodenal bulb (D1), usually on the anterior wall. Occasionally, in about 10-20% of cases, ulcers are located on both the anterior and posterior walls, and these are called 'kissing ulcers'

Endoscopic description of an ulcer should include:

- Location
- Number
- Size {using the fully opened cups of a biopsy forceps (about 5 mm in size) to estimate}
- Shape: linear, oval, round
- Edges: flat, raised
- Ulcer base, using Forrest's classification

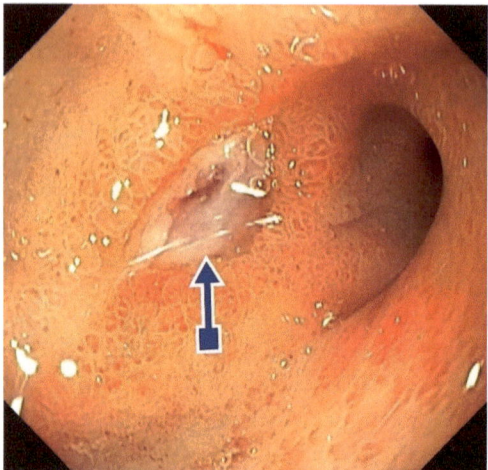

Figure 8.7: Ulcer on the anterior wall of D1

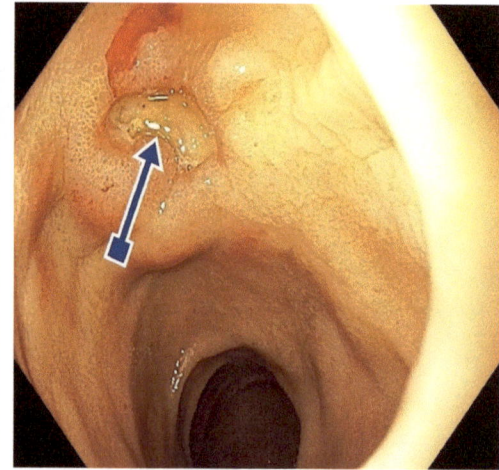

Figure 8.8: Ulcer on the superior wall of D1

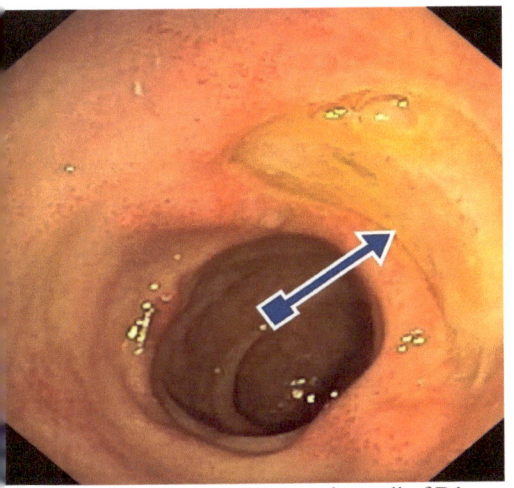

Figure 8.9: Ulcer on the posterior wall of D1

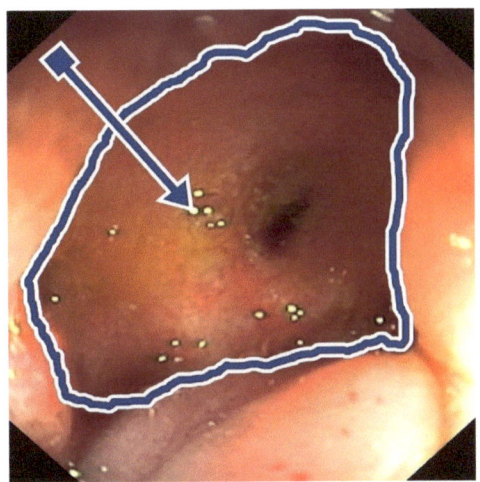

Figure 8.10

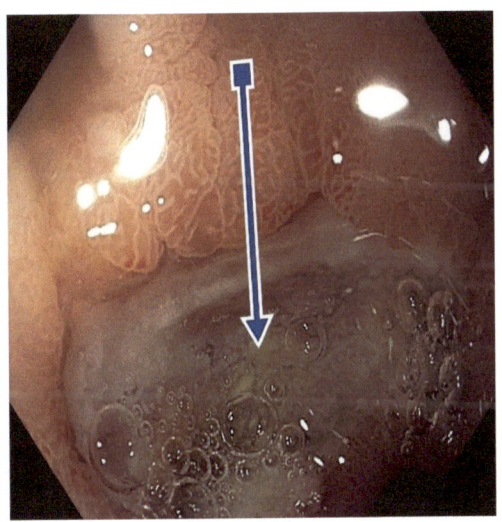

Figure 8.11

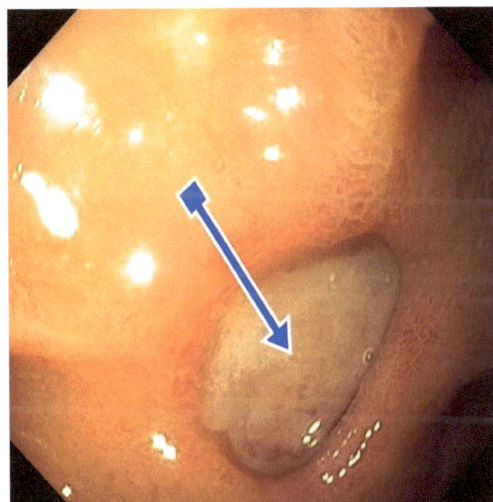

Figure 8.12

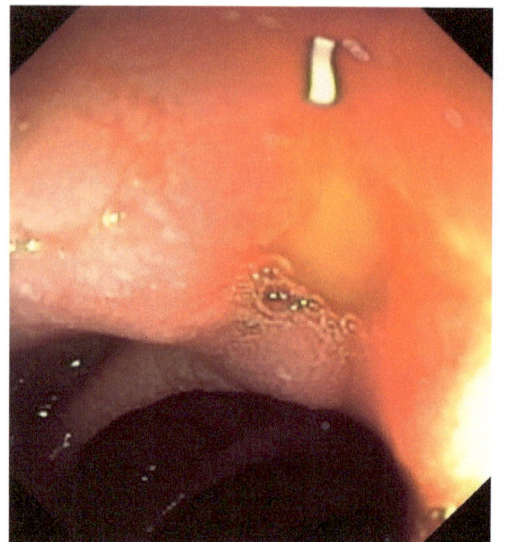

Figure 8.13

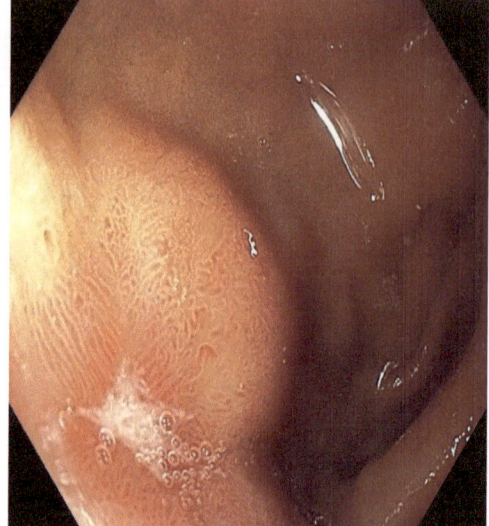

Figure 8.14

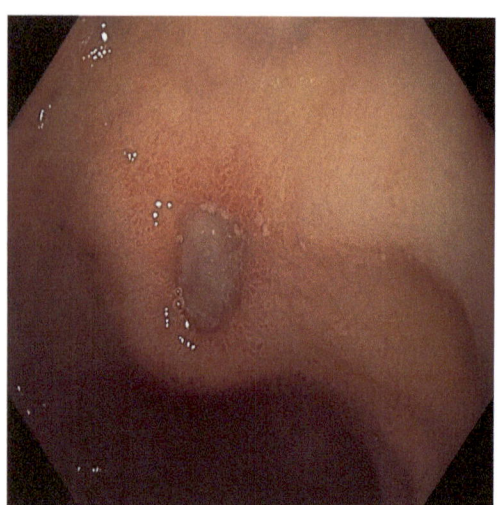

Figure 8.15

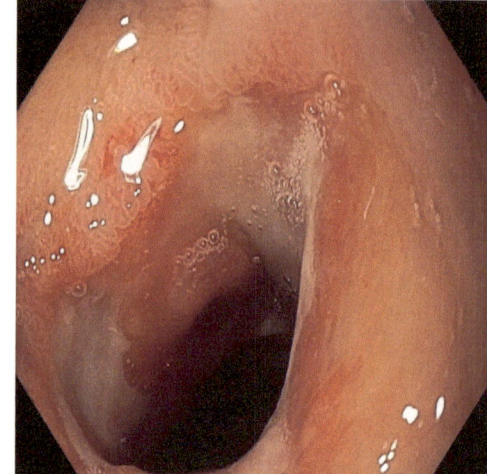

Figure 8.16

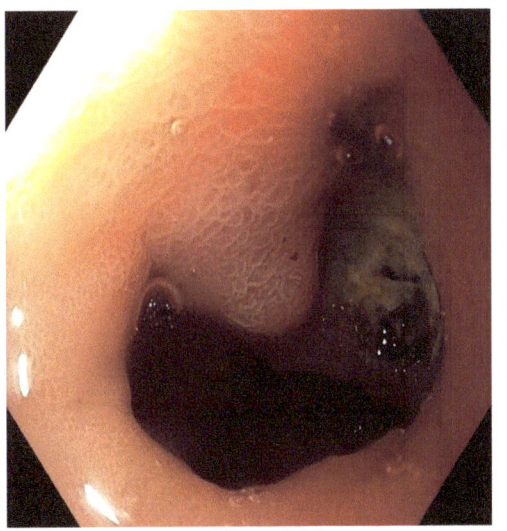

Figure 8.17

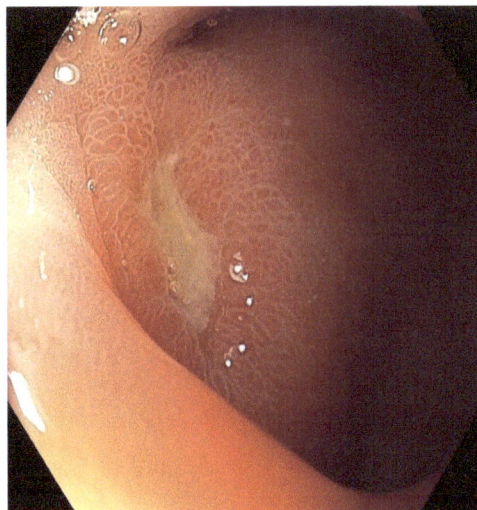

Figure 8.18

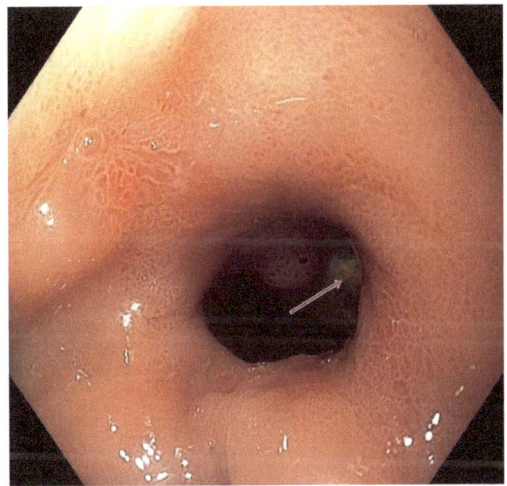

Figure 8.19

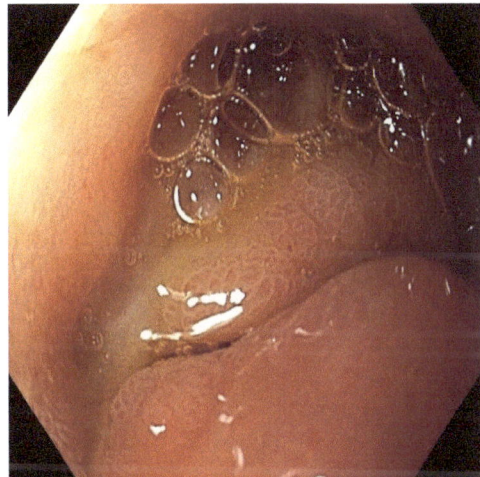

Figure 8.20

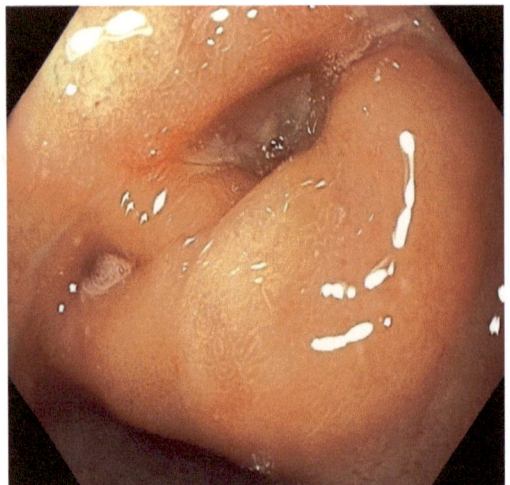

Figure 8.21

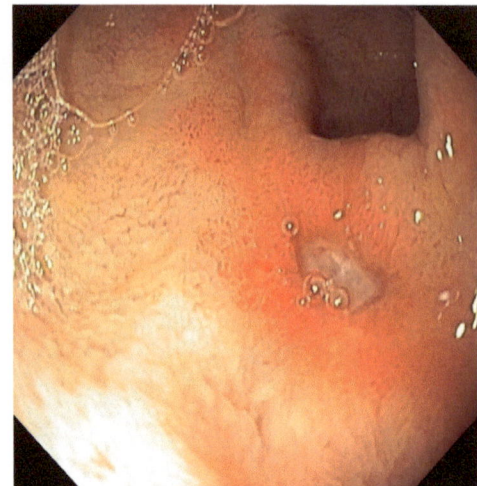

Figure 8.22

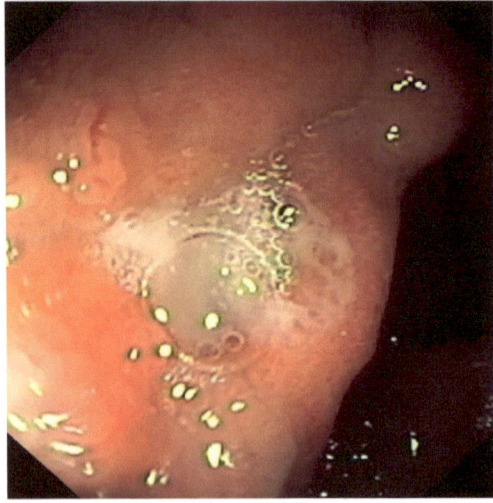

Figure 8.23

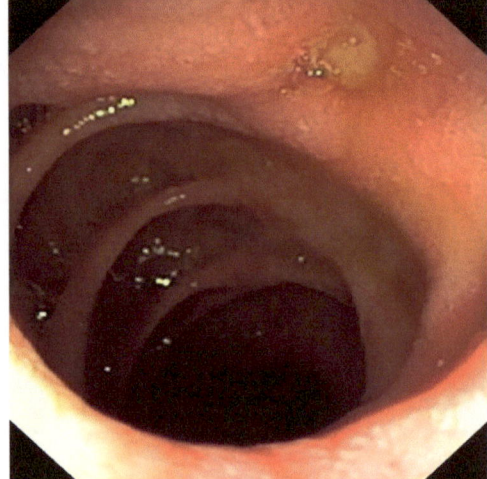

Figure 8.24

Other Duodenal Abnormalities

The following duodenal abnormalities are uncommon

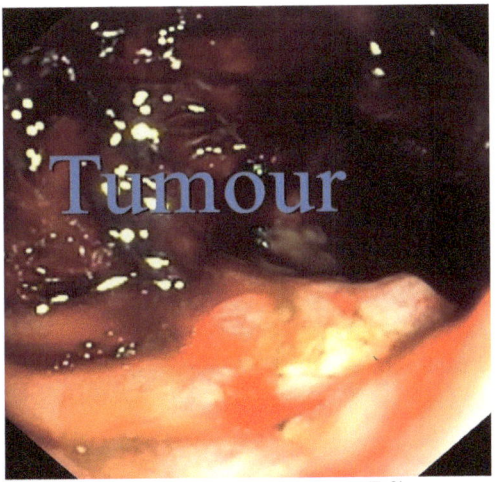

Figure 8.25: Duodenal tumour (D3)

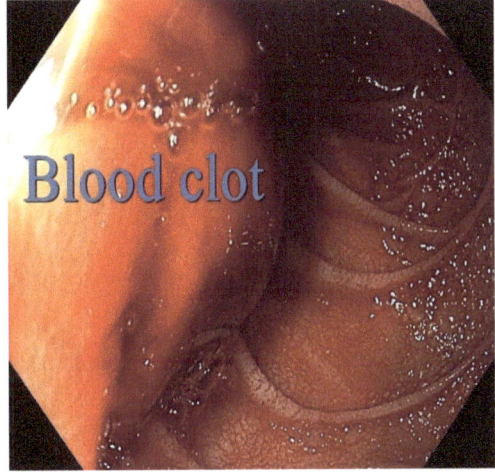

Figure 8.26: Blood clot in the duodenum (D2)

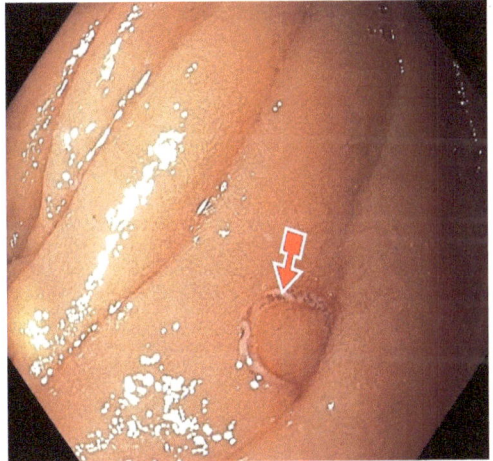

Figure 8.27: Worm in the duodenum

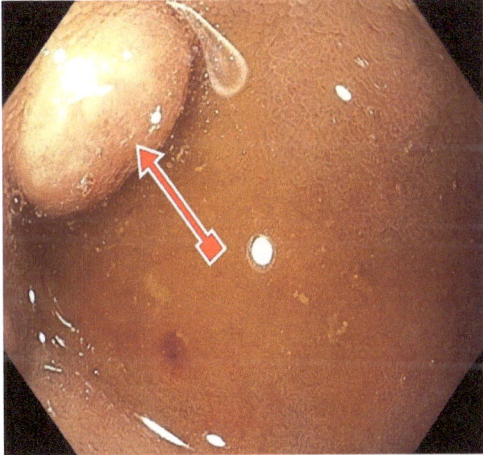

Figure 8.28: Duodenal polyp

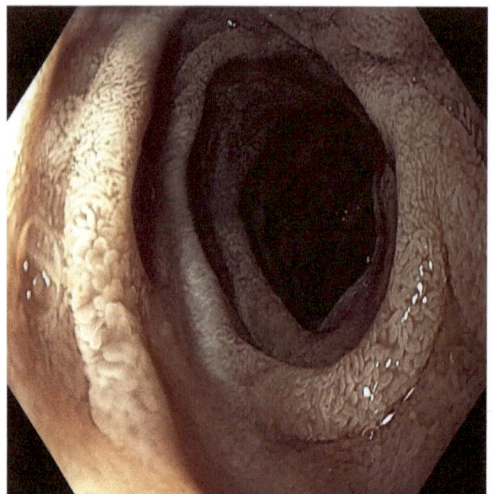
Figure 8.29: Duodenal lymphangiectasia

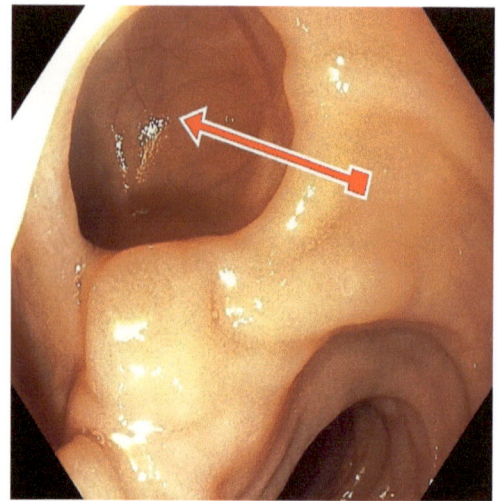
Figure 8.30: Duodenal diverticulum (D1)

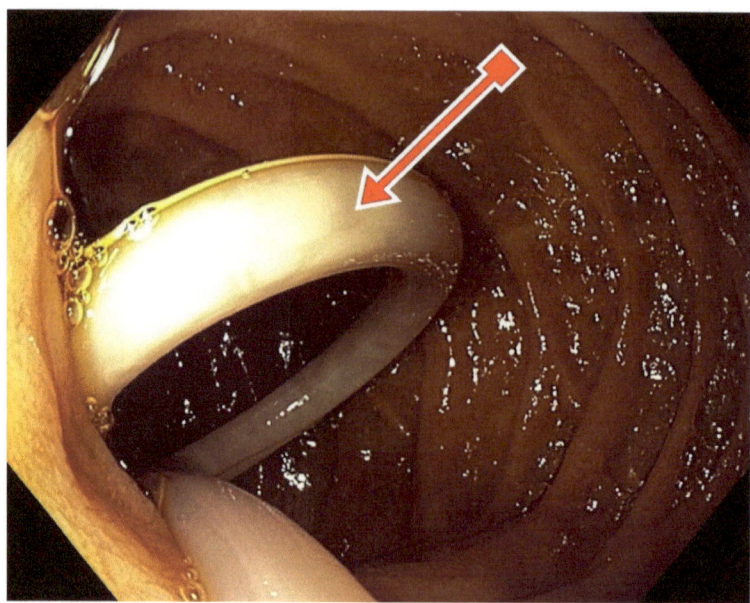
Figure 8.31: Adult *Ascaris lumbricoides* in the duodenum (D2)

References

1. Schiller KFR, Cockel R, Hunt RH, Warren BF. (2002). Atlas of Gastrointestinal Endoscopy & Related Pathology (2nd ed.) Massachusetts: Blackwell Science.
2. Block B, Schachschal G, Schmidt H. (2004). Endoscopy of the Upper Gastrointestinal Tract. New York: Thieme Stuttgart
3. Ginsberg GG, Kochman ML, Norton I, Gostout CJ. (2005). Clinical Gastrointestinal Endoscopy. China: Elsevier Saunders

www.ingramcontent.com/pod-product-compliance
Lightning Source LLC
Chambersburg PA
CBHW040221220526
45473CB00001B/75